MW00596080

FINANCIAL FITNESS

THE JOURNEY FROM WALL STREET TO BADWATER 135

William Corley

Table of Contents

DEDICATION

I dedicate this book to my mother and father. I am forever grateful for your love, never ending support, encouragement, and the example you set by always going the extra mile.

INSTRUCTIONS

How to Use Financial Fitness:
The Journey from Wall Street to Badwater 135

Each chapter in this book is divided into sections. Aside from the first chapter, which comprises three segments, each chapter contains two parts consisting of physical fitness and/or health-related tidbits, followed by information pertaining to financial well-being. The first section of each chapter will hopefully serve to motivate and enlighten you if you are considering joining a Couch to 5K program, debating trying yoga, or wondering what's in those green drinks that cost over $10 at health food stores. I like to think of life as a journey that we all travel together, comprised of our unique situations and experiences, as well as our shared paths.

I was able to get myself into shape and maintain my physical well-being for the last decade plus, which leads me to believe there's hope for everyone. My personal journey is not one of mystery and luck, but one grounded in hard work, perseverance, and resilience. It's what Angela Duckworth, Professor of Psychology at the University of Pennsylvania, calls "grit." Along the way, I have discovered that most people who accomplish great things have high grit factors. It takes grit to finish college, pursue a career, raise a family, and maintain a healthy exercise routine and diet.

The second section of each chapter chronicles my pursuit from Wall Street to entrepreneurship; it also includes concepts and steps to attain and maintain financial fitness, all of which I learned and garnered over a thirty year career in investment services and wealth management. My hope is that this section will enable you to examine your personal financial goals and create a plan, or financial road map, to achieve your financial fitness. I touch on the subjects of saving, investing, stocks and bonds, insurance, and retirement strategies. Like physical fitness, financial fitness is achieved over a lifetime of good habits, persistence, and commitment.

Financial Fitness can be read cover to cover, or by selecting the parts most appealing to the reader. In the appendix are basic nutritional guidelines and a fitness training plan. While I am not a coach, I share my own experiences and the results I achieved. I hope this reading enables you to ponder your own journey, leading to further success in your life.

"You're off to Great Places! Today is your day! Your mountain is waiting, so... get on your way!"
—Dr. Seuss

PREFACE

My intention in writing this book is to share with others the steps I have taken to attain physical and financial fitness. I detail my path from being a flat broke 20 year old kid from Tennessee to making it on Wall Street and becoming a millionaire in my late 30s. I tell the story of my transformation from being a couch potato in my early 40s to running my first 5-kilometer event and subsequently qualifying for the Boston Marathon, competing in the New York Ironman Triathlon, and a decade later racing the Badwater 135. Badwater is a non-stop, 135 mile ultra-marathon run in Death Valley, California, in the middle of July, where temperatures exceed 120 degrees; it is considered to be the "world's toughest foot race." *Financial Fitness* shares the story of how my quest to wealth and fitness unfolds.

"This could be the start of something big."
—Clarence Clemons (E Street Band)

INTRODUCTION

If I Can Make It, Anyone Can

"The secret of getting ahead is getting started."
— Mark Twain (Humorist)

According to the Census Bureau, there are approximately 7.5 billion people living on planet earth. Ten years from now the world's population is projected to grow by nearly a billion. The United States comprises 324 million residents, which is 4.4 percent of the world total. America generates $19 trillion in gross domestic product, approximating 25 percent of all economic output, ranking it number one in the world. Our population expands at the rate of one person every fifteen seconds. Each of these individuals will require goods and services their entire lives to survive. Those willing and capable of fulfilling these needs can benefit.

The median household income for Americans exceeds $56,516; this is greater than 50 times the amount earned by 4 billion of our other brothers and sisters cohabiting the planet. Being born in America is like hitting the jackpot. It offers a real chance for anyone to pursue a life of personal freedom, physical well-being, and financial independence. In many ways, I see the American way of life as self-chosen.

This book is a chronology of my personal journey towards financial independence and healthy living. Each chapter provides lessons that I've learned along my health and fitness journey, as well as tried-and-true practical advice on investing and making money. My story begins during my early workaholic days when I hardly ever exercised, my eating habits were terrible, my waist size was expanding, and my blood pressure was rising. Healthwise, I was on a crash course to nowhere, and I didn't even know it.

The premise of this book is to live life to the fullest. My definition of a fulfilled life is likely to be somewhat different than yours. The commonality amongst us is that everyone willing to put forth the effort deserves the opportunity to succeed. In *Financial Fitness*, I focus on two specific areas of life that are important to most of us: health and wealth. I wager that just about anyone can achieve remarkable results with their financial well-being and their vitality for life by making wise, calculated, logical decisions, and then going for it. By going for it, I mean setting high goals, dreaming even higher, and never settling.

Like most others, I care about people and society. I want to make a positive impact in the world around me. For that to occur, I need to be in sync with my thoughts, attitudes, actions, and reactions. I am neither a pessimist nor an optimist; I'm a pragmatist. My preference is to see the proverbial glass of life at least half-full, but I can't say that I always see it that way. There are times when I become disoriented, and my outlook is jaded. It is during the times when I feel off kilter that I slow down and focus on re-centering myself. I've learned to be open during these down-slope episodes, which often enable me to learn, deepen my understanding, and force me to pause and take the time necessary to reflect on my next steps. Throughout my journey, exercise and mindfulness have helped me shape a better version of myself and improve my outlook on life.

Financial Fitness comprises 14 chapters, each dually purposed. In the first half of each chapter, I share adventures pertaining to the world of endurance sports. I also touch on how I improved my health and the effort it required to get there. In the latter half of each chapter, I provide my viewpoint and experiential knowledge on the subject of wealth attainment and management. As a financial services veteran for over 30 years, I have provided investment insight and product selection to institutional and retail investors, managed money professionally, offered investment banking services to small companies, and founded a full-service brokerage firm.

Over the course of three decades, I have been responsible for informing and navigating investors through the ups and downs and twists and turns associated with the whims of financial markets. Professionally, I have towed the line during times of duress and extreme uncertainty. I was at my terminal manning the phones during the crash of 1987, the tech bubble burst in 2000, and the most recent housing meltdown of 2008, known as the Great Recession.

I see the topics of healthful living and wealth attainment closely related. I've witnessed first-hand that healthy living often leads to wealthy living, in more ways than one, and throughout this book, I delve deeper into this realm. I believe anything is possible if you put your mind to it. As you read about my journey, I will offer tips and insights that I learned along the way; I invite you to share your tips with me by email at chip@chipcorley.com.

CHAPTER 1:

5K: The First Few Miles

"The journey of a thousand miles begins with a single step."
— Lao Tzu

January 15, 2005 was the beginning of it all—running, that is. My son Chipper and I arrived early to run our first-ever 5-kilometer race. Chipper was 11 years old and competing in the 14 and under age group, while at 43 years old, I was in the 40 to 44 age group. The weather was 68 degrees, brisk and cool by South Florida standards, but ideal for the 5K race in which we were about to compete. By the time I pinned Chipper's bib number to his shirt and fastened on mine, it was nearing race time. There we were at John Prince Park in Lake Worth, Florida, about to compete as father and son in our first race.

I was proud of my young son for being there with me at the starting line; I also felt proud of myself. I hadn't even begun the race yet, but there was something in me that knew this was right. I began running, showing up to compete, putting myself on the line; there was an element to it that was bigger than me. In reality, this 5K race was a gateway to another place, a better place. By running this 5K competition with all of my heart, I could test my physical limits in a way I hadn't done in over 20 years. It was also an opportunity to be more of a father to Chipper. Up to this point, I was knee-deep in work. All of my efforts were focused on making

1

money. But on this particular morning, money had nothing to do with it.

I had been a mediocre athlete growing up in Tennessee. I even played third-base collegiately at Palm Beach Atlantic University — a small parochial school in West Palm Beach, Florida. Sports had always been a part of my life, and I liked the challenge of it all. But when it came to running, I had never competed in a race in my life. Ten minutes before the gun was set to go off, Chipper and I headed for the starting line. We positioned ourselves midway towards the back of the crowd. Racers were in front of us, behind us, and along both sides — we were right in the thick of it. I was nervous about Chipper potentially getting tossed around or knocked down by the hoard of runners, but I had every intention of protecting him. I thought to myself, how in the world am I about to race this race and why am I dragging my 11 year boy along with me? Chipper had complete trust that I knew what I was doing, but in reality, I was a desk jockey, and for me, participating in athletics was best summed up in front of a TV watching sports with the remote control in my hand. In all fairness, I did play golf regularly, but only with a motorized cart to drive me as close to each golf shot as possible. A moment later the *Star Spangled Banner* began to play on a boom box. I listened to our national anthem with pride. During the two minutes the music played, I drifted back to how we arrived here in the first place.

This journey began the previous summer, June to be precise. The school year had ended for the kids, and no school meant no studies, and all fun. Chipper's idea of fun amounted to playing video games day in, day out, for hours on end. He excelled at gaming and would lose himself in the entertainment of it all. Each time he started a new video undertaking, he would play it until the end. When Chipper was younger, we often played these video games together.

Now, at 11, he was far superior to me in the gaming realm. It was the second week of summer break for Chipper, and I had just gotten home from the office around 7 p.m. There was still plenty of daylight left before the summer sunset. When I went to say hello to Chipper, he was completely absorbed in the next video adventure. I thought to myself — I'm his father; am I doing anything to help him develop into the type of young man he needs to become? I hadn't taken the time to teach him some of the basic skills of working around the house, yard maintenance, or manual labor for that matter. The reason was that I didn't care for that type of work myself, and for me to teach him required me to do it. It was his mother that primarily kept him on the right track, taught him the basics, and tutored him with his homework. His sisters were involved in multiple activities, while Chipper's extra-curricular consisted of mostly playing video games.

I said to him, "Put your sneakers on son; we are going for a run."

Bruce Barber, who years later died far too young in a tragic plane crash, was a very dear friend of mine at the time. I respected the way he raised his children and the three compulsory rules he enacted for them to live by: 1) they should be decent citizens; 2) they needed to do their best in school; and 3) they must be active in sports. I had decided that I was going to adopt the same guidelines for my children. But I had slipped up on the sports portion for Chipper; I had pretty much let him do his own thing. It was all about to change that one late June evening when I told him that we were going out for a mile run. Out the door we went to the end of the driveway, and then we began running together. In no time Chipper was panting and wheezing. His physique looked healthy and normal, but his physical conditioning was non-existent. I wasn't much better myself, but I needed to set an example. From that point on, we began running regularly.

Seven months later, there we were at the starting line of the race. The gun blasted and off we went. We were running fast, relatively speaking. At mile one we were both feeling it. We had gone out with the crowd at a pace too fast for us, but we kept moving forward. Mile two was pretty much a blur, and with a mile to go, we stayed the course. At the finish line we were happy it was over. Chipper took 4th in his age group, and I ended up 16th for my age group.

Chipper stayed with running and excelled. During his senior year of high school he made it to the state finals as a mid-distance runner in both the 800 meter, and 4 x 800 meter relay.

The Entrepreneur's Journey

"I am convinced that half of what separates successful entrepreneurs from non-successful ones is pure perseverance."
— Steve Jobs (Apple Founder)

My son and I learned that it was possible to start from ground zero and work our way up to running a 5K. Starting a business possesses some of the same attributes it took to run a 5K: determination, perseverance, and commitment. For 33 years I've been active in the business world. I have worked for large and small companies alike. I have advised, funded, and founded companies across a variety of industries. As an entrepreneur my experience has been in small business. Small businesses are defined as companies with less than 500 employees, and account for 99% of all companies in America. Presently, I run a financial services firm, as well as an industrial equipment provider. I have built two profitable million-dollar companies from the ground up that I am actively working at today.

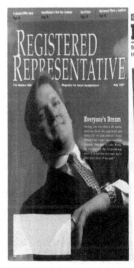
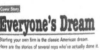
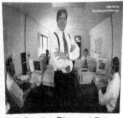

While running these companies has not always been a cakewalk,

I've learned and gained necessary experience along the way, and met great people who have inspired me.

Creating a successful business is both science and art. Businesses are not one-size fits all by any means. Circumstances, finances, experience, the economy, and changing times often dictate what works and what does not. I view each business as a unique endeavor that necessitates those involved to give whatever time, effort, and energy it takes to make the company operate effectively. It requires a deliberate mindset and one that is enduring. My entrepreneurial journey is a reflection of the things I've done seemingly successfully and unsuccessfully. There is an adage that states, a smart person learns from their mistakes and experiences, while a wise person learns from other people's mistakes and experiences. It's true; experience is derived from putting in the hours with effort, and it is wise to learn from experts. I became a millionaire at 38 years old, because I was results oriented, cared about people and their financial well-being, was unwavering in getting it right, and I wasn't afraid to work my butt off. Somehow, I landed on the cover of our industry's magazine!

People often ask me what it takes to start and run a successful small company, and if they should consider doing it themselves. My answer is, "It depends." Many people lead incredibly successful careers working for others. In today's economy, most employees function as entrepreneurs in various capacities regardless of the size of the company, or their roles. Large companies are essentially agglomerations of smaller

6

companies working in unison. Innovation and drive, the same attributes necessary to build a business, are often necessary to succeed and grow within a company, and I predict that it is going to be magnified even more in the future. It is paramount for businesses of all sizes to have employees with reasoning skills that enable them to make decisions in the company's best interest. Entrepreneurship is the organizing and operating of a business or businesses. Entrepreneurism is synonymous with risk taking. What does it take to be an entrepreneur? I believe that <u>desire</u> is the essential ingredient for choosing to go into business for ourselves. Desire leads us to the start line, gets us past those first few steps, and keeps us going. Desire is the fuel that pushes us forward when thoughts of quitting surface. Before embarking on a new enterprise, it is imperative to be clear on our goals and desires and to commit.

What was my desire? To get rich and create a work environment that was intellectually stimulating and fulfilling for me, and to do it better and smarter than the big banks. Sure, the benefits of working for someone else abound: financial stability, employee benefits, 401k matching, paid holidays, and vacation pay. Why would anyone want to leave when there's so much to lose? That is a question that everyone has to ask themselves before they take the plunge. I was money motivated. I am driven by nature. The pressure I impose on myself surpasses the pressure anyone else can put on me. Having a boss breathing down my throat on high-stress Wall Street was counter-productive. The pace

I worked at was frenetic. From the moment I sat down at my desk each day, it was full-speed ahead. I pushed myself to the max daily. Making money was a numbers game. The more calls my team and I made each day, the greater the odds of success. I had been pushing at this tempo since graduating from college in 1985. I was all work and no play.

I was one of four children from a middle class family. Like any working family, meeting expected and unexpected financial responsibilities was difficult. My father and mother worked hard their entire lives. At a young age, I decided that when I was older I was going to earn enough money so that I wouldn't have to worry about the cost of living. With my all-in at work lifestyle on Wall Street, I had little time for other aspects of my life, such as taking care of my health, let alone our family of five. I realized early on that financial success comes with sacrifices. Caffeine was the fuel that got me through long days and nights at the office. Taking the entrepreneurial leap, and walking away from the corporate world was not about what I was losing, but about what I was going to gain: freedom, a newfound sense of purpose, and a fiercer, more passionate drive than was ever possible when I was working for someone else.

Money Principles

Earning, Spending, Saving

"Those who understand interest earn it, those who don't, pay it!"
—Jack Sauder (Businessman)

When it comes to money, there are <u>three</u> principles necessary to getting it right: earning it, spending it, and saving it. The first and most important principle of the three is that we must enjoy <u>earning</u> money. If you think about how much of our life is spent going to school and then devoted to working, it is important that we are engaging our effort in something we enjoy. If we love how we are making our living, we are going to have a much more fulfilling life. The second principle we must employ pertaining to money is to enjoy <u>spending</u> it. Spending money can be simply marvelous. We can buy our loved ones' gifts, go on that ski vacation in Utah, take a European cruise, or go out to eat at a really fancy restaurant and drink the best red wine. The third principle pertaining to money is that we must enjoy <u>saving</u> it. Saving money can be equally enjoyable as it enables us to buy the things we need when we need them most. Saving money allows us to accumulate reserves in case of an emergency or a job loss. Saving money is the path to home ownership; it's what makes retirement the golden years. And the most amazing thing about saving money is that money properly invested begets more money, without us doing anything but investing it.

I wish that I had learned the principles of investing money earlier in life. Working on Wall Street and investing money for myself and others over the past 33 years, I have seen firsthand the potential earning power of invested savings. Stocks, bonds, and cash are where most people choose to invest their money. Stockholders are actual owners in the company; bondholders own the debt of the company. Stocks are considered riskier than bonds and cash. Why put your money in stocks? Stocks, also known as equities, have historically outperformed all major asset classes: real estate, bonds, gold, and the dollar. Each of these major assets has their merits, but equities have proven to be the best performers throughout history. Since I entered this business, the Dow Jones Industrial Average has grown by over 9% a year compounded, which means that every dollar invested in 1984 doubled every 8 years; $1 invested in 1984 is worth over $17 today.

As a financial consultant, I have found that no two clients are alike. Certainly, all clients want good things in life, but it is how they go about obtaining them that makes the difference. Amateur investors have been known to buy at the top and sell at the bottom. Investors are often ensnared by the hype of the media. When the portrayed experts espouse China, gold, bitcoin, IPOs, small caps, or the next hot trend, impulsive investors are apt to purchase them in their online accounts. They tend to miss the mark not so much on which investments they buy, but how they allocate all of their assets. Prudent investors allocate their capital across multiple asset categories for specific reasons. For example, institutional investors often allocate their capital across asset classes such as domestic equities, foreign equities, U.S. treasuries, inflation-protected securities, private equity, hard assets, real estate, precious metals, foreign currencies, natural resources, derivatives, alternative investments, and cash, and strategies such as absolute return, event driven, and value oriented. Successful investing comes at a price. Investing properly requires knowledge, experience, flexibility, adaptability, self-awareness, and capital.

The economy is alive and in a constant state of flux. It is either expanding or contracting at all times. The rate of economic growth, or economic slowdown, is what makes the world of personal finance replete with complicated outcomes. And no one really knows how long, or at what trajectory the prevailing trend will last. Stock market prices are leading economic indicators, meaning that if the stock market is going up the economy is apt to follow. When stocks sell-off abruptly, it may very well be an early warning sign that the economy is about to fall on hard times. Stock prices are known to lead fundamentals. So, if that is the situation (the economy is either in expansion or contraction mode at all times), a smart solution may well be to invest for both outcomes, specifically, inflation and deflation.

John F. Kennedy said, "A rising tide lifts all boats." This means that when the economy grows, everyone benefits. However, the economy can only rise so far and so fast before it needs to digest its gains. Here's how the economic cycle works. When conditions are favorable, sentiment is high and people are more willing to spend money and take more risk, resulting in elevated asset prices in housing, stocks, tips, commodities, wages, and the like. Eventually, the economy begins to overheat or an exogenous event, such as rapidly increasing oil prices, occurs. Then, the Federal Reserve begins to raise interest rates to prevent asset bubbles from developing. At this point, markets halt their advance and begin to ebb. Market behavior is driven by fear and greed, as depicted in the chart.

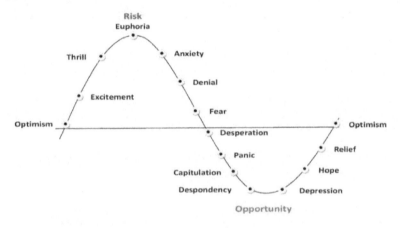

Warren Buffett said, "Only when the tide goes out do you discover who's been swimming naked." Buffet is implying that investors who have taken on too much risk are forced to sell and limit their losses as the market retreats. The adverse market reaction to this selling turns into a negative feedback loop. Newspapers, television, and the internet sensationalize that investors are losing money. At this point, investor sentiment changes from optimism to pessimism. Fearful investors and consumers start tightening their belts, cutting back on their discretionary spending and risk taking, and in turn, upending the economy and sending it into recession. During this period of retrenchment, the Federal Reserve lowers interest rates to restart the economy's growth engine. Bond prices move inversely with interest rates; when rates fall, bond prices rise. During rate easing cycles, bonds, especially U.S. treasuries, are a profitable place to be.

Money itself is like the economy in that it is constantly in a state of perpetual motion. Money is like a seesaw teetering from risk-on, to risk-off. Whenever there is fear or pessimism in the economy, money will shift to risk-off. And what that means is that money will shift out of the stock market and into the bond market, primarily U.S. treasuries. Immediately, investors earn interest on their treasury bonds and are no longer subject to economic uncertainty. Investing one's assets for multiple scenarios, such as inflation or deflation, boom or bust, euphoria or despair, is what I call win-win investing. Self-awareness is the catalyst that makes it all possible.

CHAPTER 2:

Yoga

The Gateway to Healthier Living

"So whether you do your first downward dog at age 14 or 44, it is not your history, but your presence on the mat that counts."
— *Pattabhi Jois*

It was May of 2004, a day like any other day as far as my health was concerned. I was scheduled for my annual check-up with Dr. Raj Khambhati, MD. For as long as I could remember, I never liked going to the doctor's office. I always felt doctors were in a position to deliver unwanted news. After the initial routine of weighing in, blood work, and other samples, along with measuring my blood pressure, Dr. Khambhati spoke right up, "Your blood pressure is too high. You have hypertension." He explained that the risks associated with hypertension could be either a stroke or heart failure. I felt a jolt in my stomach. "What does this mean for me?" I asked. He was reserved in his prognosis and asked if I was under more stress than normal. I didn't think so, but thought about the question for a moment.

For the past two decades, I had been working as a stockbroker in the fast-paced world of finance. Investing money for others can be unnerving. The reasoning was straightforward — if I recommended to a client that they should invest $25,000 into Coca-Cola stock and let's say, two weeks later, Coca-Cola reported quarterly results that were below street consensus, sending the stock price tumbling by 15%, well, I can tell you the client that took my recommendation wasn't very happy. Making matters worse, the way I was wired, I couldn't seem to let go of the Coca-Cola trade, and I berated myself for picking it in the first place. Now, I was being asked if I was under more stress than usual. I told my doctor that I didn't think so. Dr. Khambhati wrote out a prescription for 180 milligrams of Diovan and instructed me to have it filled promptly and take the medicine twice a day. In a state of disillusion, I asked Dr. Khambhati how long I would have to take the 180 milligrams of Diovan. "For the rest of your life," he said.

One thing was certain: I needed to improve my health. Sure, I had started running, but obviously, I needed something more, something to slow me down and help me to achieve tranquility. I started researching alternative forms of exercise and decided to give yoga a shot. Practicing yoga was completely unfamiliar to me. I didn't even know anyone that had ever done yoga. The only thing I could recall about yoga were the crass stereotypes I'd heard growing up, such as why would anyone want to put their legs behind their heads and who are these crazy people chanting "Om." None of this dissuaded me; I was always willing to try something new. Yoga, I presumed, was a combination of suppleness and calmness, and I was lacking in both, not to mention flexibility, which I knew was key for overall fitness. I was stiff as a board. The idea of bending over and touching my fingers to the floor was a laughing matter. I was like the tin man in *The Wizard of Oz* without any oil. If yoga could help my flexibility to improve and offer a meditative element, I was open to it.

I decided to try out hot yoga for my first yoga class due to its convenient location. Cheryl was my yoga instructor and the owner of the studio. She informed me that I would be practicing the hatha method of yoga and that I would perform 26 different poses in a room heated to over 100 degrees. She told me that I needed a towel and sufficient water to manage the heat and to get through the postures. After changing into my gym shorts, I entered the yoga room. The heat hit me in the face and the first thing I thought was get on the floor—heat rises. I began to panic. Bad decision. This place was an inferno. The very idea that I could do anything besides sit on my mat was beyond my scope of reason. Immediately, I thought about leaving the place altogether, but my health issue convinced me to stick around. The 90-minute class started promptly at 4:30 p.m. Cheryl indicated that it was important for me to stay in the heated room for the entire class. I was convinced I was going to die. She said that if I needed to rest, I could lie down on my yoga mat, but leaving was frowned upon. Great.

When class started, the athletic spirit in me jumped right into it. I was breathing, bending, stretching, and sweating. The front of the room was completely mirrored, enabling each of us to see ourselves. There I was in the mirror attempting the postures. I hoped no one noticed me. Cheryl was strict about when to drink

16

water; she would tell us when we were allowed to drink. My water bottle was right there. I was dying of thirst. When she gave the go ahead to drink, I gulped down half the bottle. By this time my shirt was soaked, and I decided to take it off. There I was standing in front of the mirror looking over 40 years old, analyzing myself along with the other male yogi practitioners. A few of these guys looked like they modeled for *Men's Fitness,* most of the others resembled my middle-aged physique and there were still others that looked even worse. If they could do this hot yoga, I assured myself that I could, too. Oh, I should add that for every man in the room practicing yoga, there were at least ten women right alongside us. That was both good and bad. On the one hand, practicing yoga next to some of Boca Raton's top lady yogis had its plusses. On the other hand, trying to do these awkward postures in front of these women was ego-deflating. These female yogis exemplified strength, grace, and splendor with every movement. Conversely, I was clumsy, flabby, and out of my element.

If it weren't for the fact that there were other people in the room doing these postures, I would not have thought it was possible. Each minute was taking forever to pass. I didn't know how I was going to survive. It was the most strenuous activity I had ever done in my life. My only lifeline during that initial hot yoga class was my water. I drank it like my existence depended on it. As a first timer, Cheryl guided me through each yoga pose; each one of the 26 was difficult for me. It was one posture after another, 45 minutes standing up, with 35 minutes on the mat, and the last

10 minutes resting in the shavasana pose, which consisted of lying flat on my back. I felt as if my body was being stretched on a stretching machine. Hatha yoga was torture. Finally, Cheryl said, "Rest in shavasana." I couldn't believe that I had made it. I immediately fell asleep for a few minutes—passed out is more like it. I had completed my first yoga class. I had no idea how I survived. I waited until just about everyone left the room before I gathered my mat, towel, water bottle, and shirt, and wearily moved towards the men's dressing room. I cautiously entered the shower, clothes and all, turned the water to cold only, and just stood there leaning against the wall as the cool water worked its magic; it took a while for me to acclimate.

After finishing up my shower, I slowly got dressed and gathered my belongings. Cheryl met me as I neared the door and I asked her if I could buy another cold bottle of water. She asked me how I was feeling and what I thought of my first yoga class. I was starting to come to my senses and I told her that I felt pretty good. She invited me to come back again soon, and I assured her that I would. By the time I started driving off in my car, I was feeling better and better. I gulped down that bottle of water and stopped at the store to purchase Gatorade. Drinking that orange Gatorade was pure ecstasy. By the time I finished it, I was a new man. My skin was glowing, my head was crystal clear, my energy level totally modulated, and I felt serene. The hot yoga took every ounce of will I could muster to complete in those 90 minutes, but I did it and felt rejuvenated. From that moment forward, I was prepared to make yoga a part of my life.

Mentorship Matters

"Tell me and I forget, teach me and I may remember, involve me and I learn."
— Ben Franklin

Self-awareness to me is the ability to accurately perceive reality. Self-awareness is the mirror that reflects our internal selves. Personal finance is not the subject that comes to mind when one discusses the positive attributes of yoga, but in many ways the two disciplines actually go hand-in-hand. Yoga is a pathway to self-awareness. It is through self-awareness that we are best able to preserve and improve ourselves. Self-awareness is an intuitive flood light that informs us and warns us of potential outcomes, and it is also the spotlight to guide us along our internal path. Self-awareness in yoga is one of the stepping stones that leads to further personal understanding, discipline, flexibility, and adaptability.

We all have wants, needs, hopes and dreams; to fulfill these aspirations requires a certain level of financial security and financial independence. I believe strongly that anyone practicing self-awareness in their financial affairs is destined for success. Self-awareness is that internal voice that guides us each step of the way and enables us to make the best decisions for our lives. That's not to say we have to make all the decisions, quite the contrary. Generally, there are mentors in every field that can help us to find answers to our questions. For example, it is logical for us to hire the services of an established architect if we want to build a dream home. The same applies to someone aspiring to make films for a living. Apprentice film makers need to obtain the proper education and learn all they can about producing a movie from an expert in the field. We see this occur every day in sports — elite athletes train with elite coaches. Accomplished artists learn from accomplished art instructors. Wherever there is a model student, there is a model teacher. I call each of these facilitators mentors. When it comes to getting a leg up, mentorship matters!

In business, as in life, everyone needs mentors. It is a privilege for anyone to have a proven expert as a guide in all capacities. A mentor is a seasoned, successful, sage adviser. Mentorship is the integration of someone else's knowledge and know-how. Mentorship is empowerment. The best mentors are usually very busy people. Mentors are not going to do "it" for us, but they will provide insight. I have benefitted greatly from my mentors personally, professionally, and physically.

As a professional money manager, my mentor is Sam Stovall, The Maven of Manhattan. Sam is one of the most sought after investment strategists on Wall Street. I am fortunate to dine with Sam several times a year. During these meetings, I am able to openly share my views with a true expert in the field of finance. Sam in turn assists me in examining my own ideas and often introduces something new about the financial markets that I've yet to discover. Over the years we have developed a close friendship, and to me, friendship, like fine wine, gets better with age.

For many years, I engaged the services of Dr. Arnold Pusar as my life coach. Dr. Pusar, a Board Certified Clinical Psychologist, is the wisest man I've ever known. His brilliance, life experiences, and insightfulness contributed immensely to my personal transformation. Life in many ways is a mystery. It can be complicated and overwhelming at times. People often try finding the answers to their dilemmas in all the wrong places. Logic would say that if my best thinking and choices got me into this mess, why would that same thinking be best in resolving it? It wouldn't. There are psychologists and analysts whose primary purpose is to address our unresolved issues. Finding an expert in the field of human development and behavior to help figure out life challenges is a sound bet. Through self-awareness and the right mentors, it's possible to thrive and keep one's affairs in order.

CHAPTER 3:

Half-Marathon - I Think I Can

"Structure is not just a means to a solution.
It is also a principle and a passion."
— Marcel Breuer (Architect)

The sound of my alarm awoke me from a deep sleep on the 29th of January at 3:15 a.m. It was just over a year since I had run my first 5K with my son, and now I was about to try my hand at the half-marathon distance—13.1 miles. The race was scheduled to begin at 6 a.m., with start line access opening at 5 a.m. The drive to Miami would take me an hour and I didn't want to rush. I had driven down the day before to pick up my race number and timing chip. The race was set to begin in front of the American Airlines Arena, home of the Miami Heat. Driving down on race-day morning, my mind was pensive. I had never run more than 9 miles. Now I was about to attempt 13.1.

For the past 12 months, I had been running on a regular basis. I had even joined the local running club for their 6 a.m. runs on Sunday mornings. The first time I showed up at the Winn Dixie parking lot at 5:45 a.m. to run with the group it was pitch black out. I had no idea what I was about to get myself into. My head was spinning. How many miles was I going to run? Would I even be able to keep up? I was excited to begin running, but nervous that I would not be able to hold the pace of the other runners. Everyone was talking amongst themselves. I didn't know a soul.

Getting up early that first Sunday morning to go run was very difficult for me, because for the past 20 years, I had enjoyed staying up late on Saturday nights. But there I was, the wannabe runner, sleep deprived, and standing alongside veteran runners who were complete strangers to me, about to hit the road. Before I knew it, the group was off and running. My first reaction was trepidation; my breathing was labored by the intensity of the pace. I had no clue which direction I was going, and if, or when, I would ever catch my breath. *Stop*, my lungs screamed. *Abort mission*!

I could not believe the predicament I was in. I needed oxygen, not to mention that my legs were malfunctioning. Was I supposed to tell these strangers around me that I was redlining? I had positioned myself in what I thought would be a safe place near the back of the pack with the slower runners. I miscalculated; they all ran as a unit—fast, medium, and slow, males and females all ran together. There was no dispersion. So, there I was running with these experienced runners hanging on for dear life. In reality, I could have stepped aside and gathered myself at any time, but the athlete inside of me would not let me. My pride was at stake. I would have rather kneeled over and died on the spot than to cry out in agony. My lungs felt like I'd been running for an eternity, but my watch told a different reality: it had been just a few minutes.

When we reached mile three, everyone started slowing up and then they all out stopped to refill their water bottles at a makeshift hydration station, which consisted of a utility bucket full of bottled water and Gatorade. I could not believe that we had actually stopped. I had expended energy that I did not know was in me, and was completely exhausted. The group held up for a few minutes. They were all in high spirits. While I was standing there one of the runners asked me how far I was planning on going. I said I wasn't sure. I had no idea where I was or how I would find my way back. He informed me that the runners would be going various distances, ranging from 7 to 20 miles, and if I chose to run with the group, I just had to follow them. However, if I wanted, I could take a shortcut straight back on the road in front of us that would take me back to where we started; it was about two miles. I thanked him, but said I had previous commitments requiring me to turn back. In reality, the only commitment I had was to find a way out of this self-induced flogging. The idea of running another four miles with these athletes would have been impossible. After the runners took off again, I went back to the hydration bucket to quench my thirst. It was still dark as I began the two mile jaunt back to my car. After walking for a few minutes, I tried jogging, but I had nothing left in me.

For reasons unknown, I began showing up to run with the group every Sunday. Even though I was no early bird, I found getting up and joining the experienced runners made the miles go by faster. As I became more consistent with running, I began to learn from others how they had evolved. After each run, the runners that showed up that morning would hang out for a few minutes and talk about that morning's run. I would listen attentively to what each runner had to say and ask questions to improve my running skills. During one of these after run pow-wows, I spoke with the top runner in the group, Jon Pagalilanuan (Jon P.). In my eyes, Jon was a mythical character. "Your fitness level is not measured by how far or fast each training workout is; fitness is measured by how fast you recover," he said. His insight was beyond my scope at the time, but I took it to heart. From the onset, I continuously raised the bar for myself. Weekly, I attempted to increase my speed, the distance of my long run, and my overall total weekly running mileage. My pace was just over 11 minutes per mile for a 6 to 7 mile long run at the time. During the week my total mileage was around 20. Up to this point, I had no idea where this new found sport of running was taking me.

My first running breakthrough came from a pair of Brooks Adrenalin running shoes. Up to this point, I had pretty much winged every step of my running, and I'd been running in sneakers I purchased on sale. To me, all running shoes were pretty much the same, so I had not given it a second thought. My lack of knowledge and ignorance as a runner pretty much rejected the idea that finding the right running shoes mattered. The very thought I could find a shoe that actually made my feet happy was wishful thinking. From the moment I put the Brooks on, they felt terrific. As a runner, finding the right sneakers is like finding a pot of gold. The running shoe immediately felt comfortable and durable, with adequate support. From the moment I laced them up, my confidence soared. I believe the first step to begin running is to try on as many running shoes as possible until you find a pair that feels great on your feet. I ran in Brooks for the next five years.

The half-marathon. It came up on me all too quick! After parking my car and figuring out my bearings, I headed to the starting corrals. People were everywhere. Helicopters were flying overhead and news reporters were televising it all. There was a certain energy in the air that made me excited. Ever since I was a young boy, the moments leading up to an athletic event caused my stomach to do flip flops. Normally, I am talkative, but right before I am ready to compete I shut down and become quiet. The opening ceremony got underway at 5:45 a.m. with the city's bigwigs welcoming everyone and the playing of the national anthem. The athletes with disabilities started the race. Ten minutes later, the field of full and half-marathoners took off running down Biscayne Boulevard.

There we were, thousands of runners on the MacArthur Causeway watching the sun rise each step of the way. At mile four, we arrived at the world famous South Beach. As we ran along Ocean Drive, there were no cars to be seen; the route had been closed to traffic for the race. It was surreal. Before I knew it, I was passing mile nine. I was in unchartered waters from that point onward. Every running stride was further than I had ever run before. At mile 11, I was hurting and wanted to give up. At mile 12, the anticipation of being close to done set in. When I arrived at the final turn on Flagler Street, I sprinted the best I could for the final 150 meters. And just like that, it was over. I had officially completed a half-marathon. 13.1 miles in 2:08:22. I finished 2,251 places behind the winner.

Structure + Focus = Confidence

"The most important thing is to focus."
— Lei Jun (Billionaire)

What did I learn from the training and eventual completion of the half marathon? Running those early Sunday mornings, putting in the miles, and pushing myself beyond my limits were getting me somewhere. I was encountering a better version of myself, peeling away my doubts, and introducing an element of confidence that I hadn't known I lacked. Belief in myself, along with my training, enabled me to push past the doubt and fear and move toward the finish line. How does that relate to personal finance? The structure, focus, and confidence that I gained via running are analogous to what it takes to become an effective investor.

To achieve financial fitness, it is necessary to employ structure, adopt healthy financial habits, and commit to the journey. If I invested my money wisely in stocks, bonds, cash, and real estate, then, on an impulse, I decided to purchase an expensive car or boat, much of the progress that I had made could be lost as a result of this impetuous act. How does one keep from derailing? I believe that everyone should have a financial plan or roadmap. A roadmap enables you to plot your course, measure progress, and establish long-term goals. I prefer a roadmap because I can visualize it better in my mind, instead of the image of a written plan.

Structure

What's structure have to do with it? Structure has everything to do with it. When it comes to my own financial plan, my primary focus is to earn more money than I spend. In the early days of starting my business, I often had to take on additional work—beyond my full-time job—for that to be a reality. Saving for an emergency fund is also critical. At the onset, my goal was to have three months of savings set aside so that I could cover my living expenses, if necessary. In addition to earning more than I spent and establishing an emergency fund, I have always been diligent about organizing my monthly expenses—mortgage, gas, food, utilities, insurance, car payment, and later, tuition for my children's education. By planning out my expenses, I am clear on exactly how much I need to earn on a monthly basis, and aim to budget more in the event of unexpected repairs or bills.

Individuals choosing to work for themselves should scrutinize every single purchase for their business and do whatever is necessary to limit expenses. When I first started out, I lived with three others in a two bedroom apartment to save money. At the time, I focused only on my needs: not on my wants. Now, in terms of structure my key criteria are organization, consistency, and focus. Organization enables me to stay on track on a daily basis; consistency keeps me moving forward on a personal and professional level; focus enables me to execute and accomplish my business and personal goals.

Healthy Habits

Financial structure is the foundation to healthier money habits. I am a firm believer that the healthiest financial habit involves saving more and spending less. If you know you're going to need a new car in the coming year, save for it. If you want to go on a vacation, plan accordingly. My healthy habits are derived from my core values. In order for me to maintain healthy habits, I have to ask myself what's most important to me: family, friends, health, wealth, and play. In that context, my financial structure consists of planning, protecting, and investing. If I break it down, it looks something like this:

Prepare	**Life is a journey: be prepared.**
Protect	**Better to be safe than sorry: insure.**
Invest	**Compounding growth is powerful: invest now.**

There are lots of possibilities for those seeking creative ways to save or earn money. Online Apps, such as Acorn and Robo Advisor, make the process for those just starting to invest into the stock market quite easy. Those looking to earn extra income by selling merchandise may choose online consignment shops or auction sites such as eBay and Etsy. If you have a creative side, explore the various artsy outlets on the internet that enable you to sell your goods online. Being part of a carpool or driving a car for Uber, Lyft, or Amazon are ways to earn money part-time. In the appendix section, I list websites, apps, and money saving solutions that can immediately make a financial impact.

Investing for retirement is critical for your future financial well-being. Remember to fund your retirement plan on a yearly basis; those who are not self-employed should consult with the company's human resources department to learn more about health, life, disability and other benefits, and be sure to explore any company retirement plans, such as a traditional or Roth 401k.

Commitment

Like all long-term plans, the key is to commit. Know what you seek in the long term, and tweak your plans as necessary throughout your career. Sure, we all fall off track now and then — a splurge on that one item you really want—but it's up to you to get back on track. I advocate revisiting your plans and reminding yourself about your long-term goals on a quarterly basis. If you want to retire early, it will require a lot of saving throughout your career. Commit to your goals; make them your way of life; adapt when necessary. When I finished that first half-marathon, it made me wonder what else I could possibly achieve if I put in the time, energy, and focus. As soon as I hit one of my financial goals, I ponder over how I can reach higher goals, and make a commitment to obtain them.

CHAPTER 4:

Triathlon - Try Anything

*"Until you face your fears, you don't move
to the other side, where you find the power."*
— *Mark Allen (Ironman 6x Champion)*

During an early morning run a few months after my half-marathon, I asked Jon P., "Where do we go from here?" All of this training was stimulating, but I wondered when it ended. Weren't we supposed to back it down at a point and take some well-deserved leisure time? His answer was simply, "It's a way of life." I looked at him with utter bewilderment. For the past six months, I had been pushing myself, constantly increasing my mileage, and now someone had just told me that I would basically be on this road to perdition forever. Sure, I felt clear and alive after putting in a vigorous run, but it was never easy. For me, running wasn't a way of life, yet.

Fast forward a few weeks later, when my athletic juices started flowing at the idea of entering a multi-discipline race. I was reading *Men's Health* and there was an article about short distance triathlons. I read the article thoroughly and was in awe that men and women alike were competing in a race that encompassed swimming, biking, and running. Outside of an occasional snorkeling outing or an infrequent scuba diving trip, I could not recall the last time I swam. The idea of competing in a triathlon was a stretch of my imagination. I had a beach cruiser parked in my garage (with two flat tires from non-usage), which pretty much summed up my current state of biking. For the most part, I had not ridden a bike in years. I felt confident about the running leg of the race, but even then, I had never run immediately after biking and swimming. As I began contemplating the idea of what it would take for me to participate in a triathlon, I was filled with anxiety. At the same time, I visualized a larger than life image of myself if by chance I actually completed a race entailing a swim, bike, and run. Certainly, there were a lot of triathletes in Florida and across the nation that competed in these events; I just never thought at this stage of my life I would be one of them.

One of the benefits of living in South Florida is that I can participate in outdoor sports year-round. As fate would have it, a local sprint triathlon race was coming up in April, less than a month away. I remember how anxious I felt once I decided to sign up and give this multi-discipline race a shot. I was concerned about how I was going to manage the waves during the ocean swim. I thought about the biking segment of the race, followed by the run. I even contemplated how embarrassing it would be to finish in last place. Although nothing in my life depended on this triathlon, I was still afraid of failing. From the moment I signed up, time was of the essence. There wasn't a minute to spare; it was vital for me to get into a swimming pool, start practicing, and develop a semblance of confidence.

Days later, I joined the local YMCA and began swimming in their Olympic-sized pool. I incorporated three swim sessions a week into my schedule. I was a certified lifeguard in college, so at one time in my life I was an above average swimmer, but that was a long time ago. My skill had dwindled. As a side note, during this period my youngest daughter, Julia, launched her swimming career. Julia joined the area's top program and dedicated herself to swimming and spent her youth in the pool six days a week. Julia's hard work paid off. She became an elite swimmer, collegiate athlete, and a champion mid-distance runner to boot (proud Dad plug).

The sprint triathlon consisted of ¼ mile swim, 10-mile bike, and 3.1 mile run. I knew that once I got to the run portion of the race, I would be okay. The swim on the other hand, which would be in the Atlantic Ocean with its two to three foot surf, was out of my comfort zone. As for the biking portion of the triathlon, I was just going to wing-it. Initially, I contemplated buying myself a new bike, but I held off. Why was I going to spend money on a new bike when chances were that I might never ride it again? Up to now, when it came to getting in shape, my track record was pathetic. Instead, I borrowed a friend's Raleigh hybrid 10-speed for the race and decided I would think about buying a new bike in the future, if I actually finished the race and still had any interest.

Race day

The triathlon was set to start at 7 a.m. We were required to have our bikes placed in the designated transition area by 6 a.m., accompanied by our cycling shoes, helmets, food, and water. Immediately after getting my things situated, I hurried to the men's restroom. I had to wait in a long line that didn't seem to move. As I stood there, I started to panic, heart racing and all. I watched the seconds pass by on my watch. I couldn't believe how long each person was taking to finish their business in there. Each minute that passed was one minute closer to the race beginning. It seemed unimaginable to me that I was going to miss the start of the race because of nature's calling. Then finally, it was my turn. Relief swept over me. I was overjoyed I hadn't missed the race start. Running barefoot with my swim goggles and cap in my hand, I hustled to the beach where the swim portion of the race was about to begin.

There I was, standing at the edge of the shore with hundreds of other triathletes about to run into the ocean full of waves that I had no idea if I could navigate or not. I remember

RACE-DAY CHECKLIST: What to bring to every event

GENERAL
- ☐ USAT membership card
- ☐ Photo ID
- ☐ Registration confirmation
- ☐ Directions to venue
- ☐ Course map
- ☐ Money
- ☐ Race uniform
- ☐ Race numbers and timing chip
- ☐ Sunscreen
- ☐ Sunglasses
- ☐ Anti-chafing product
- ☐ Extra clothes
- ☐ Watch

TRANSITION GEAR
- ☐ Towel(s)/Transition mat
- ☐ Water bottle(s)
- ☐ Gels/energy bars and drinks/salt tablets

Never worry about forgetting important items again. Use this checklist to ensure you arrive at your next race relaxed and prepared.

SWIM GEAR
- ☐ Wetsuit
- ☐ Swim cap
- ☐ Goggles

BIKE GEAR
- ☐ Bike
- ☐ Helmet
- ☐ Bike shoes
- ☐ Bike gloves
- ☐ Tire pump
- ☐ Spare tube(s)
- ☐ CO2 cartridges
- ☐ Tools
- ☐ Bar-end plugs

RUN GEAR
- ☐ Running shoes
- ☐ Hat/visor
- ☐ Race number belt
- ☐ Socks

PERSONAL REMINDERS
_____
_____
_____
_____
_____
_____
_____
_____
_____

USA TRIATHLON

asking myself, what am I doing here? In the seconds prior to race start, I contemplated the fact that I was in way over my head. I thought about quietly walking back to my car and writing this whole thing off as a bad idea.

Bang! The gun went off and just like that I went into the roaring Atlantic seas. I immediately went out as fast as I could. Why, I will never know. My experience up to this point was in aerobic distance running and there I was sprinting, anaerobically out to where the water was deep enough to swim. Once I started swimming—drowning was more like it—I was gasping for air. I could not catch my breath, and my heart rate was through the roof. I should add that during those tense moments other swimmers were crashing into me and hitting me with their hands and feet. I felt like I was fighting for my life out there. This all happened in a flash. My survival instinct was to stabilize my breathing, and to do this I changed from swimming freestyle to the breast stroke. Within a minute or so my heart rate normalized, and I was breathing properly. I switched back to the freestyle stroke and battled onward. The waves were rocking me up, down, and sideways. I was trying my best not to swallow water, but each time an unsuspecting wave hit me in the face, I invariably gulped sea water. I dug deep, and before long I was swimming back towards the shoreline. Once the water was shallow enough for me to touch my feet on the bottom and stand-up, I knew the hardest part for me was over. Relief washed over me.

As soon as I stepped foot on the beach, I began running. Once again, I went too fast, causing me to lose my breath. After I slowed down a bit and got myself back under control, I made my way to the bike area. By the time I entered the bike transition zone, most of the bikes were already gone. I took my time removing the sand from my feet and putting on my running shoes. Most of the bikers wore cycling shoes, but my bike had pedals, and so I sported sneakers. I was actually glad I did not have to change shoes again later. Off I went, still wet from the ocean, but feeling accomplished that the swim was behind me.

Riding the bike parallel to the ocean coast was amazing. The morning air felt cool and exhilarating against my wet trunks and body. I was taking it all in. The bike route was a switchback, enabling slower athletes to see the leaders on their return to the transition area. Watching the elite cyclists zoom past me was amazing. I was enthralled that I was actually participating in an event with the fittest athletes in town. I pushed hard on my hybrid bike; it seemed as though I had to peddle twice as much to equal the output of bikes built for triathlons. It did not faze me one iota. To me, my bike was a rocket that was allowing me to be part of one of the most incredible events of my life. Before I knew it, the 10-mile bike ride was completed.

Now it was time for me to run, and I was ready. My legs felt spongy at first and were not responding as expected. I panicked for a minute at the thought that I would not be able to run properly. Instead of running, I felt like I was affecting a slow jog. At mile 1, my legs came back to me, and as they did, my running speed increased. From that point on, I began passing other triathletes ahead of me. Each time I passed someone, it lifted my spirits. Competing in my first triathlon was epoch. I only had two goals: to finish the race, and not to come in last place. Mission accomplished.

If at first you don't succeed, try again.

"The impediment to action advances action.
What stands in the way becomes the way."
—Marcus Aurelius (Emperor of Rome)

While my try-anything attitude proved successful in the sports arena, it wasn't always the case in my professional life. Some of my business ventures did not go as planned. This is where my newfound athletic training was proving helpful: I was aware that if I wanted to improve, I needed to change the way I was doing things, create a strategy, and execute.

In 2002, I acquired a mid-sized stock brokerage firm in San Francisco that was presented to me by my friend and executive, Dolores Strauss. For the next four years, I commuted from Florida to California on a monthly basis to oversee business operations, clean up the problems, and cement relationships. At the onset, the acquisition brought me the quick growth that I sought. By 2006, because of technological changes in the industry, we were finding it nearly impossible to increase revenue. As a mid-sized company in the financial services space, we did not have sufficient capital, technology, or human resources to compete with the better equipped financial super powers. As CEO, it was my job to oversee the management team, lead by example, and figure out how to increase our company's profits.

Profitability was key, but equally important was the firm's limited investable capital on the balance sheet. The firm's fixed-income desk was an essential part of our trading operations. This division generated a meaningful share of revenue, but required a considerable amount of capital to fund customer buy and sell orders. Allocating funds for growth purposes would diminish our capital base and consequently, leave our trading desk shorthanded of needed capital. In order for the company to succeed and flourish, it had to grow. Unfortunately, growth consumed cash, and if we spent cash in one area, we would find ourselves with a shortfall elsewhere. It was a catch-22. At one point, we increased our marketing and advertising expenditures with the intention of increasing sales, but our endeavor proved futile. Every financial journal, newspaper, website, and television station was overloaded with financial ads, rendering our attempt to capture new business in vain.

The financial services industry is personal and high-touch. Licensed professionals are the lifeblood of the business. In order to execute orders and counsel clients, it is necessary to be licensed. Licensing requires studying for and passing challenging examinations, all of which can take months to complete. This made it difficult to hire licensed professionals in a timely manner, and yet without these licensed financial advisors on staff, we couldn't generate sales.

Beyond that, to succeed we needed our licensed financial advisors to be producers and top talent. That meant competing against the likes of Morgan Stanley, Merrill Lynch, and Goldman Sachs, which was nearly impossible. The larger firms would offer six and even seven figure upfront signing bonuses for proven producers to join their companies. We did not have the resources to compete. Up to this point, our success strategy was to grow by making acquisitions of smaller financial services companies. The tricky part with acquisitions as a growth strategy is that it does not resolve the dilemma of insufficient organic growth. For many months, we lingered and stagnated until it became imperative to make changes.

We had a staff of over 30 employees that serviced 200 brokers and 5,000 clients. It may sound like a lot, but we could have handled double that amount. In fact, we did not have enough work to keep everyone busy, and the firm's profitability was being drawn into question. We had no other choice but to cut overhead and eliminate excess personnel. As with any company, downsizing created its own moral hazard. Instantly, employees began to wonder when or if they would be let go. Morale hit rock bottom. Management worried that key personnel might jump ship if they thought the company was having difficulties. And the financial advisors, who were managing clients and producing revenue for the firm, started asking lots of questions. Holding it all together was a juggling act.

Capitalism is said to be "the perennial gale of creative destruction." What this means is that the competition will always be fierce and will never let up. Succeeding in business, more so today than at any point in history, is a game of survival of the fittest. 90 percent of all new business ventures fail within the first five years and 90 percent of those remaining fail in the next five years. So, why chance it when the odds of making it were stacked against me? That is where participating in the sprint triathlon gave me that extra oomph I needed to press on and not give up. By putting myself out there and taking the risk during that race, I evolved. I became more than I had been, and was able to make decisions that I previously could not. I believe humans are built to go for it and that self-worth is a byproduct of effort and achievement. I've found the more challenging a goal is to accomplish, the more rewarding it is. I believe that each day has its own unique ebb and flow divinely packaged as life itself. And as long as I stay open and aware to what is happening inside and outside of me, things always work out as they should.

CHAPTER 5:

New York Marathon

"Never underestimate the power of dreams and the influence of the human spirit. We are all the same in this notion: The potential for greatness lives within each of us."
—*Wilma Rudolph (Olympian)*

In January 2006, I submitted my application for entry into the New York City Marathon. I had never run a marathon before and really did not think I could, but I applied just the same. Tens of thousands of us hopeful runners applied via the lottery system, each hoping that our application would be selected to run the prestigious 26.2 miles throughout New York City's five boroughs. Wilma Rudolph, former world-record holder and three-time Olympic gold medalist, was from my hometown of Clarksville, Tennessee. I revered her unprecedented athletic accomplishments. As a fellow Clarksvillian, I visualized running the marathon and being part of my town's unquenchable athletic spirit. If I were to be accepted into the New York Marathon, I was determined to give it my all. The odds of winning a slot in the race by lottery were approximately 1 out of 10. As chance would have it, I won a slot.

From the moment the email arrived saying that I was one of the 37,000 runners selected to participate in the race, I was in awe. I felt a mix of thrill and trepidation. I was elated at the thought of being a part of the most famous marathon in the world, while at the same time I was angst-ridden. I had no idea how a 20-year desk jockey like me could ever run a marathon. News travels fast in the running community, and within minutes I found out that several of my closest running friends also received admittance confirmation. At first, I wasn't sure if I should tell anyone that I got in. I was superstitious to acknowledge that I was about to take on something that stretched beyond the scope of my abilities. The furthest I had ever run was 13.1 miles, and that had crushed me. Now I was entertaining the idea of 26.2 miles. It had me unhinged.

Everyone in my immediate family was excited and proud of me for even attempting this undertaking, and I appreciated their encouragement. When it came to anything sports oriented, my father was always my biggest fan and support. From the time I was a young boy in Tennessee, he coached me in football and baseball. As I grew up, he attended every sporting event I played in, even when I sat the bench. My dad would be there in the grandstands, watching the game attentively if by chance I got to play. On those rare occasions, he and I discussed every detail of my efforts on the field. My dad shared in my joys and sorrows. He let me be the rambunctious teenager I was while growing up, and loved me unconditionally. His belief in me was paramount to the success I attained in business and the man I was becoming. I'm not saying my dad was perfect; he wasn't. He was short-tempered. But whenever I needed him to be there for me, he was. I couldn't wait to tell him the news, as I knew he would be proud of me. I called him on his cell phone and he immediately answered in his usual positive manner. He knew how busy I had become in the fast-paced world of finance and was happy whenever I called. I told him right away that I was going to be running the New York Marathon. He said, "Son, that's incredible."

After speaking with my father, I felt settled. I knew instinctively that to make this race happen for me would require having a game plan. I began analyzing marathon training schedules for beginners online. I identified several that were highly regarded and I chose one that seemed right for me. I decided on a 20-week training schedule that would have me running 20 miles a week to start and incrementally building up to a peak of 50 miles a week. Even though I had been running for over a year at this point, my body resisted it when I stepped up either my mileage quantity or intensity. If I ran too fast during a track workout or logged excess miles beyond my usual amount, my ankles and calves ached and my body took more days than normal to recover. It was at this point in my running pursuit that I began to learn to keep training even when I was sore, worn out, and slightly injured. It was in the grit that the growth occurred.

Participating in the New York Marathon was beyond the scope of any athletic undertaking I had ever imagined. The planning overwhelmed me at the onset. I had to map out hours in the day to train, figure out what to eat and drink during the race, learn about hydration, find running shoes that could get me through longer distances pain free, and figure out which socks worked best for me, too. The list in my head was exhaustive. To tackle it, I opted to break it all down into smaller segments. Next, I established and set priorities from that day forward until the actual race day, November 5th, which was one day shy of my 45th birthday. Priority number one was to complete all scheduled training runs to the best of my ability. I approached training like it was a job.

My training schedule consisted of running five times per week. Three of the runs were very difficult for me: Wednesday's track repeats, Thursday's tempo run, and the weekend long run, where I increased the length of mileage almost every week. I was a model student when it came to following the game plan. No matter what was going on in my life, I made training part of it. I would run at whatever time fit into my schedule on a given day, albeit morning, afternoon, or evening. I knew if I completed the schedule to the best of my ability, I would be prepared for the race. I worked in a high-rise office building in downtown West Palm Beach, Florida. At times, my work obligations botched my running plans. To compensate for the unexpected interruptions, I often ran in the middle of my work day. I would change into my running clothes in my office, then sneak out the back door without telling anyone, and go run for an hour. When I returned back to the office, I was drenched in sweat. I went straight into the men's room, cleaned up, and changed back into my work attire without anyone ever knowing I was missing. Running the New York City Marathon was important to me. Training purposefully was essential for me to reach my goal of finishing the race in less than 4 hours, which would require me to maintain a 9:09 pace—a speed faster than I had run in my prior half-marathon. Three weeks before race day, I ran a long training run that was more like a dress rehearsal for the marathon — 20 miles with 14 of the miles at a 9:09 pace. It was difficult, but I held the pace and made it. I was ready for my first marathon.

Marathon 26.2

The night before the marathon, I had trouble winding down and sleeping. It was uncomfortably hot in my room and yet the temperature outside was in the mid 30-degree range. I tossed and turned until my alarm went off at 3:20 a.m., with a backup telephone call from the hotel at 3:30 a.m. I had to catch a bus at 5 a.m. to transport me to the pre-start staging area. By the time I arrived at the marathon waiting area by the Verrazano Bridge, I was exhausted and a wreck. Everyone around me was excited and in good spirits. My friends were all upbeat. My pal Steve would be racing the marathon with me, but I was overwhelmed by it all and having a mood. I had a couple of hours to rest and wait before the race would begin. Clad in a

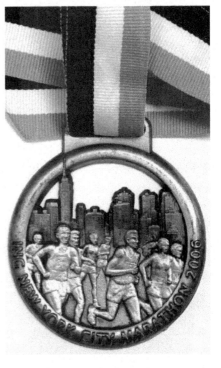

garbage bag to keep warm, I laid on the ground and fell asleep for a while. When I awoke, I felt somewhat better.

As we made our way to the race start, I was totally focused. Thousands of runners surrounded me in every direction. Once the race began, there was a 10 minute lag between the runners at the start and way in the back of the pack where I was corralled. And just like that, I was crossing the Verrazano Bridge, participating in the New York City Marathon. The experience was surreal. There were over one million spectators lining the roadways. Every single mile, complete strangers cheered me on. I felt like I was a famous rock star. We ran all five boroughs of New York City: Staten Island, Brooklyn, Queens, the Bronx, and at mile 16 crossed the Queensboro Bridge into Manhattan. The fan support was absolutely electrifying. I was completely uplifted as I entered into the city, even though I still had 10 miles remaining: miles 19, 20, 21 running through Harlem; mile 22 down Fifth Avenue; and mile 23 leading into Central Park. With just over three miles to go, I bonked. To bonk means to hit a wall, to have nothing left to offer. I was a physical, mental, and emotional wasteland. I had run the race with all of my might. My goal of sub-4 hours was in reach, as long as I kept moving and did not walk.

With two miles to go, I was fading. My mind was pushing me onward, but my legs were so sore and tired that I was finding it nearly impossible to keep running. The last mile was a blur. I was yelling out to the bystanders, "How much further?" I heard more than once, "You're almost there," but I was having trouble believing them. Minutes later I could see the 26-mile marker up ahead. I had almost made it. But then, no, I was wrong. It was a cruel joke. I had .2 tenths of a mile left and it was uphill in and through Central Park. It was the longest 300 yards of my life. When I crossed the finish line, I could no longer feel my frozen feet. I was shaking in the frigid November weather. I moaned to myself. Warmth seemed like a faraway dream. Then it began to set in. I finished. I had pushed myself harder and further than at any point in my life. I had just run the New York City Marathon, without walking at all, in 3 hours and 51 minutes. When I called my dad later to share my accomplishment, I wept.

Breaking the Debt Cycle

The rich rules over the poor,
and the borrower becomes the lenders slave.
—Proverbs 22:7

I wanted to run the New York City marathon, finish it, and come in with a decent finishing time. Knowing what was at the end of that road for me, I was willing to put in the time, effort, and energy. Just as the NYC marathon was a distant dream for me, what I learned from creating a plan and sticking to it was that tackling a goal was about 1) structure 2) hard work 3) consistency and 4) desire. Structure is the blue print of how and what I need to do; hard work is my commitment to accept and focus on the task at hand; consistency is my determination to keep at it; and desire is the hunger that keeps me moving forward. In the end, all of the structure, hard work, and consistency come down to how badly I want it. Mastery of even one of these four principles can be a real game changer; a collective mastery of each of them is the recipe that transforms dreams into reality.

In my line of business, I speak to individuals on a daily basis about their financial well-being. Debt, health care, housing, and retirement top the list in terms of financial stressors. The consensus is clear: everyone wants to be debt free, with good health coverage, a roof over their head, and live prosperously. The question most often raised is should an individual or family focus on saving, or paying off debt. The answer is both. For example, when young working professionals come to me burdened with debt, they want to know what the best steps are for them to move forward. Should they aggressively pay off loans, save toward an emergency fund, or invest? The answer to the question depends upon the debt to income ratio. If the person or family's debt payment each month is over 20% of their after-tax monthly earned income, immediate action is necessary. By that I mean they need to consider one of the following: refinance their debt, aggressively start paying down the loan, find a higher paying job, or take on an additional work to pay down the obligation. If the debt to income ratio is lower than 20% after-tax, I would advise them to keep making monthly payments, but to save, too. And saving may mean investing in a company 401k, a stock portfolio, or a savings account.

In my own life…planning, principles and purpose were keys to keeping my financial affairs in order. I learned early on the shortfalls of living beyond my means and the perils of taking on debt, particularly excessive consumer debt. Credit card companies began to solicit me for unsecured lines of credit before I even had a job. I accepted the credit card offers—my thought process was that a credit card would come in handy if I had a financial emergency.

The first time I used the card was the summer of my senior year in college. I had been hired for the summer as an insurance agent. While I was driving out of town to meet prospects, my car broke down. I pulled off the road and was able to park in the K-Mart shopping plaza parking lot. Making it to my appointments was critical if I wanted to keep my job. I considered my options, used my credit card to purchase the parts and tools I needed, and began to work on my car myself. I was relieved that I was able to fix it. I did not have the money to pay an auto-mechanic and by changing the spark plugs myself in the parking lot, my car worked properly. I remember entering the bathroom in K-Mart to clean my grease-ridden hands. I could not show up at my scheduled appointments filthy dirty. I ended up using my t-shirt to scrub off the black grime. I made it to my appointments and earned $500 on a sale—enough to cover my credit card bill, and have some extra cash, too.

Getting ahead financially was a bi-product of my learning to live within my means. From my first decent car (a pre-owned 300D Mercedes), to our first house (a 2-bedroom bungalow), I kept a close eye on the monthly outflow. I purchased our first house, a pre-foreclosure listing for $50,000. Prior to owning, I was paying $525 a month in rent. After purchasing our home, the mortgage payment was under $400. Plus, as a home owner, I was now allowed a tax deduction on the mortgage interest and a homestead property tax exclusion, which lowered the net expense even more. I had significantly less stress by being true to myself, and not trying to keep up with the Joneses. I learned to manage my monthly overhead effectively. In turn, I was able to save money for the future, and five years later, we sold the property for a profit and purchased an even nicer home.

I'm often asked which is better, buying a house or investing in the stock market. The answer is, it depends. Individuals from affluent backgrounds may have multiple choices that fit their needs. But for most folks who find it necessary to bootstrap their way along financially, I say buy the home first. As a 30-year stock market investor, I've observed that most people are far more uncomfortable when it comes to losing money than they are at making money. Rule #1 for investing is *do not lose money.* Historically, stocks have outperformed most asset classes over the long term. But now, expert economists and market strategists are forecasting slower growth in the years to come. Slower growth means fewer profits by corporations and lower returns for shareholders. A dwelling on the other hand is something that everyone needs, and by owning, you no longer have to pay annual rental increases from your hard earned money to the landlord; instead, you are paying money to yourself by building equity in your home.

Assess your current situation. Ask, how much money am I earning? What are my expenditures? How much do I spend on needs such as loan payments and rent, compared to wants such as Starbucks, movies, sports, entertainment, or the latest electronics? Write it down or put it into your computer and ponder where you are financially now and where you want to be in the next month, three months, six months, one year and three years. If you have a significant amount of debt, be it student loans or credit-card debt, it is important to be honest with yourself about how much you owe. List out your creditors and what you owe to each one. Review your loan documentation or credit card agreement to understand your minimum payment obligations. Figure out a) how long it will take you to be debt free, and b) how much interest you will have paid over that period. And then, sit down and structure a plan that will get you debt free in a reasonable amount of time. Remember that it's structure, hard work, consistency, and desire that will get you to the finish line.

CHAPTER 6:

Marathon Mania: What's Next Syndrome

Prove yourself, to yourself.
—Unknown

Completing the New York Marathon in less than four hours had been an obsession. Prior to running the race, I had scheduled an appointment with a cardiologist who conducted a full battery of tests on my heart, after which he informed me that my heart was strong and healthy. I had managed to tackle my blood pressure issue over time with regular, weekly yoga classes, running, and healthier eating. I went into the race with all the confidence I needed and achieved the goals I had set. I enjoyed basking in the triumph of it all in the subsequent weeks, until what's next syndrome set in.

My determination for that first marathon in November was beyond me. I had pushed my body to its limits those 26.2 miles. In the days following the race, it was painful to walk. I tried running after a week, but my energy level was non-existent, and my legs felt like Jell-O. By week three, I was feeling much better. I thought a lot about what I had accomplished, and that I was the first in my family to ever finish a marathon. I was proud of my race, and yet I was questioning myself — did it really happen? Did I run the NYC Marathon? Was I now a marathoner? Or, was this a one-time deal for me? Could I ever do it again? It was still fresh in my mind how unbearable those last five miles were. The thought of trying it again seemed impossible. So, there I was, skeptical and looking for a way to reconcile my disbelief. The only way for me to confront this internal unrest was to prove to myself that I could do it again. With that, I signed-up for my second marathon attempt—the Miami Marathon, to be held on January 28th, just 84 days after my first. I wanted to own the title of marathoner, but for me to believe that I truly was one, I needed to do it again. In a perfect world, I wanted not only to finish my second marathon, but to also run it in under four hours.

I was already in marathon shape per my preparation for New York, so getting ready for the Miami race was mostly about maintaining my conditioning. For the next two months, I ran and trained diligently. The ongoing running was challenging physically, and mentally. I had no idea how to keep my body whole, let alone attempt another marathon, but it was about to happen. Before I knew it, I was once again standing in front of the Miami Heat auditorium with thousands of other runners, waiting to begin the Miami Marathon.

Bang! The race was underway. I was calm and uncertain at the same time. I knew trying to run my second marathon was going to be tough. From the onset, I locked into my natural stride and pace. My game plan was simple: try to maintain a consistent pace and then hold on for dear life towards the end. I did just that. Fortunately, heavy cloud cover kept the temperature in check for over half of the race, but at mile 17 the sun came out and brought with it sweltering heat and high humidity. As the clouds disappeared, the sun's rays heated up. The temperature was rising by the mile. Living in South Florida, I had often trained in similar conditions, but never for more than 10 miles. It is much easier to run in colder temperatures because the heart does not have to work as hard to cool the body down. So, there I was, grinding it out in the heat, trying to stay hydrated, as well as taking in essential calories. Somehow the miles were passing by. With two miles to go and my heart rate elevated, I was wilting away. Any tenacity that I normally possessed was fading rapidly. As I was slogging around a turn all alone, a spectator shouted out to me.

"Hang in there, you are doing amazing!" he said.

I looked up at him, my eyes blurring. "I am?"

"Yes! You have less than two miles to go and if you hold-on until the end, you will break four hours."

How did he know that I wanted to finish this race in less than four hours? Was this man a guardian angel? His recognition and support lifted my spirits immediately. When he was communicating with me, no one else was around. He was out there enthusiastically pressing me to give it my all. A complete stranger pulling for me was all the motivation I needed to gut out those last miles. I crossed the finish line in 3 hours and 57 minutes. The experience of finishing that race, reaching my goals, and doing it in 90-degree temperatures, was inconceivable. As I made the one-hour drive back to my home, I contemplated what I had just accomplished. It didn't seem possible to me that I had just run another 26.2 miles. It was then that I knew I was a marathoner.

Qualifying for the Boston Marathon

Over the next 18 months, my training advanced. I continued to participate in local area races. As my conditioning improved, my skill level progressed. I now set my sights on the Boston Marathon. Boston is the world's oldest marathon, and it is the most prestigious of them all. The Boston Marathon fields the best runners in the world. You must qualify to be eligible to compete in the race. Qualifying standards are stringent and very difficult to meet. Qualifying times are handicapped according to gender and age. Younger runners have faster qualifying times; older runners have slower qualifying times. As a 46-year-old male, I needed to run a 3:30 marathon to qualify for my age group. That would require me running an 8-minute pace for 26.2 miles, which was faster than I had ever run. I knew the undertaking would take me to my personal edge.

I signed up for the Portland Marathon to be run in Oregon on October 5, 2008. I had every intention of giving this Boston qualifying attempt my best shot, but if I fell short, I could squeeze in another marathon attempt before the end of the year. World-Class Athlete Sonja Friend-Uhl became my first running coach. Sonja's training regimen was intense and demanding. I trained diligently for the next six months. My running mileage averaged over 50 miles a week. By the time October rolled around, I was ready to race.

I flew to Portland on Friday, two days prior to the race start on Sunday. I felt strong and ready in every way, except for my feet. I had developed plantar fasciitis, one of the most common causes of heel pain, and my feet were hurting badly. The pain I felt pre-race in Portland was the worst yet. I called my running coach Sonja for advice. Sonja advised me to soak my feet in ice and water for 10 minutes in, then 10 minutes out, twice a day until Sunday. I didn't have a bucket, so I used the waste basket in my hotel room. I filled it up with ice water and soaked my feet as instructed. The pain from the ice penetrating my aching feet was about an 8 on a scale of 1 to 10. I watched the seconds tick towards 10 minutes; it seemed like an eternity. I repeated this treatment up to race time, and I was pleased that it worked. My feet felt much better. Now, the only thing holding me back was my nerves. I was anxious as I stood at the starting line of the Portland Marathon.

The race started under cloudy skies with a slight drizzle; it felt good. I was resolute about this race. I wanted to qualify for Boston. My goal was to run precisely at the 8-minute pace and to remain focused all 26.2 miles. Mile after mile, the race went as planned. I was focused and determined. I never deviated from my pace, and when I felt myself fading, I kept pushing to my personal edge and beyond. It's amazing how the mind can turn off when the body takes over. With one mile to go, I was holding on by a thread. I needed to run 8 more minutes at the 8-minute pace to make it. I did it! I finished the marathon with a time of 3 hours, 29 minutes and 51 seconds. I met my Boston qualifying goal by 9 seconds. It was a dream come true.

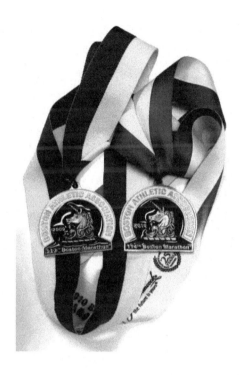

Sticking with It

"Cause when the going gets tough...the tough get going!"
—Bluto (Animal House)

What does training for and running marathons have to do with investing in the stock 'market? Everything. Training, consistency, persistence, and performance are the essentials to success when it comes to running. If you don't put in the time and effort, you cannot expect to perform well once the race starts. Winning in the stock market is no different. It takes commitment and persistence to perform well when it comes to investing, as well as a plan that adapts to each person's financial status over the years. At the onset, though, investing in the stock market requires saving and investing regularly. "How do I make a lot of money in the stock market?" is one of the questions that I am most frequently asked. The answer is multifaceted: becoming a skillful investor or money maker is a lifelong pursuit that requires commitment and patience.

In a handful of recent books, including Malcolm Gladwell's *Outliers*, Geoff Colvin's *Talent is Overrated,* and Daniel Coyle's *The Talent Code*, each author suggests that the formula to mastery is massive amounts of effort. In *Outliers* Gladwell asserts that it takes 10,000 hours of exertion in a specific field or activity to become an expert, which means that deliberately practicing an endeavor 40 hours a week for at least five years is the time commitment required to become a maven. During this training period an interested student's skill level is incrementally enhanced by applying every means available: coaches, mentors, financial journals, books, research reports, economic data, Federal Reserve announcements, blogs, periodicals, videos, illustrations, seminars, computers, even gadgets. Therein lies the answer to winning big in the stock market. But every investor has an equal chance to accumulate small wins. On Wall Street, I learned a quote that resonated: "An investment in knowledge pays the best interest."

For illustration purposes, I am going to describe three different investors, their profiles and financial positions, and what I deem to be a favorable strategy for each individual to obtain fruitful results from investing in today's market.

Investor #1: Saving $1,000

When I graduated from college, I was flat broke. I had earned a degree in business administration, but instantly figured out that a bachelor's degree was no ticket to the easy life. I was naïve, carefree, and optimistic. My first job out of college I was hired as a stockbroker trainee for a two-bit brokerage firm out of Rochester. It was run by well-dressed, hard driving Italians from New York. As a Tennessean, I was unaccustomed to the swagger and bravado that brokers, particularly the sales managers, exhibited. After studying for months and completing my Series 7 license, I was immediately put on the phone. My job as a broker trainee was to make 300 cold calls a day and generate interested prospects. It was purely a numbers game, the more calls I made, the more results I got. The environment was known in those days as a boiler room. The name was derived from the intensity of work and the pressure to make sales. I was on straight commission, so I only earned money if and when I closed a deal.

In those first few months, I barely scraped by. I literally had $3 a day to spend on sustenance. I ate bologna sandwiches, peanut butter and jelly sandwiches, or angel-hair pasta (which I called spaghetti) with olive oil, a small bag of chips, and a soda for lunch. For dinner, we had a one-hour break at 5 p.m. and would wolf down our food and then go back to work afterwards until 9 p.m. Most nights, I would go to an upscale happy hour restaurant with my friend Todd Breen where we ate gourmet chicken wings for free. We ordered a beer for a dollar and then discreetly ate wings, carrot sticks and celery until we were full. In the months to follow, the immense workload paid off, and I went from zero to $5,000 in my brokerage account. Things were looking up; it was then that I made my first investment. I had been introduced by one of my colleagues to a fella that worked for a major brokerage house with an esteemed reputation. Allegedly, this well-to-do chap was in the know. He informed me of a certain stock that was about to double in a week. He said that he would let me in on the tip if I purchased the stock through his trader. I let him know that $5,000 was my life savings and he assured me that it would soon be worth much more. I did as he instructed. As fate would have it, I lost 90% of my savings in 5 days. I was devastated. To make matters worse, I owed the IRS taxes on the wages I had earned and the bad investment left me with only $500 to my name. I learned an invaluable lesson from that loss that benefitted me immeasurably in the years to follow: do not act impetuously, and beware of lurching scoundrels.

Now that we have my early day's missteps out of the way, here is how you can make money over time in the stock market. If you are just starting out, the first thing you should do is to save up a thousand dollars in a bank savings account. Think of this money as your pot-of-gold. Each time you make a deposit into this savings account, the pot-of-gold gets bigger. This is your personal treasure chest. At the moment, it may be meager, but it won't be for long. The next step is to build a 3-month prudent reserve. By that, I mean to save enough money to pay all of your bills for 90 days without working. But I only want you to put half of your savings toward the prudent reserve account while you are accumulating the 3-months total, and I want you to invest the remaining half into stocks and bonds. There are firms today that allow investors to open an account with low minimums. Technology has driven the costs down significantly for new investors. I've taken the liberty to vet several of today's innovative firms that are making positive steps forward for newbie investors:

- Acorns allows you to invest your spare change into the stock and bond markets. It provides a great way to put small sums of money to work before the money gets spent in other ways, especially on inessentials. Acorns mobile app enables you to invest into a variety of investments anytime and anywhere.

- Betterment and Wealthfront are two leading hi-tech based brokerage houses that automate the tasks of portfolio construction and management. Both companies utilize algorithms to automate the process of asset allocation. They are known as robo-advisor or robots that replace activities performed by humans. By using technology, they minimized the cost of traditional advisors and make it possible for an investor just starting out to invest like the affluent.

These providers offer minimal deposit requirements to get started. When I say invest into the stock market, you may choose among various indices, such as the S&P 500 Index. The S&P 500 is comprised of the top companies in the world: Apple, AT&T, Home Depot, Disney, Facebook, Amazon, Exxon, and Microsoft are some of the blue chip names that investors own in the index. Not only will your portfolio be full of amazing businesses comprised of brilliant management teams, deep-rooted global footprints, and superior capital structures, but history is also on your side. Since 1928 the S&P 500 has been profitable 64 out of 88 years, or 72% of the time. Sure, there have been years when the market generated sizeable losses, but that is not the norm. There are fear mongers that incite the general public with doom and gloom scenarios. They say that Wall Street is corrupt and the stock market is a rigged casino. I'm not going to spend time debating emotions. Instead, I am going to assert that if the market is like a Las Vegas casino, then it is the investors that are the "house" with the historical odds in their favor 72% of the time.

Wise investors diversify their investments across various asset groups. Investors whose objective is growth may want to consider buying an S&P 500 Index. Those interested in capital preservation may want to add investment grade corporate and taxable municipal bonds with intermediate durations to their portfolios. Treasury Inflation-Protected Securities are U.S. Treasuries whose principal rises during inflationary periods. For those seeking specific asset allocations based on their objectives, consider consulting a financial advisor.

Investor #2: Accumulating $100,000

How did I reach the $100,000 mark? I was 29 years old and had moved to New York to work for a boutique Wall Street investment banking firm; it was a dream come true. For the past five years I had continued working long hours and my income was above average. The cost of living in New York was a big step up compared to Florida, even though my earnings were increasing. As the saying goes, "If you can make it in New York, you can make it anywhere." Let me tell you what that statement means to me. Coming from Tennessee, I learned that the only way for me to get ahead was to work hard. I was willing to tackle anything in front of me, and give it my best effort to earn money. My parents and their parents worked all their lives—hard work didn't scare me. In Florida, where I began my career working as a stockbroker, I prided myself on being one of the most steadfast workers in my office; I was totally focused. When it came to work intensity, New Yorkers play at another level. Wall Street brokerage houses redline the efforts of their sales force every single day. Everyone is measured by their monthly production totals. If you had a great month in commission, the pressure was on to repeat it in the month that followed. I could not believe how hard these New Yorkers worked; Manhattan is where I really learned how to step up my game.

As a Wall Street broker, my job at the firm was to closely monitor a handful of stocks every day. I kept abreast of each company's news releases, financials, insider transactions, stock-price movement, volume changes and the like. If there was a big move up or down in any of the stocks I covered, I was on top of it. I had built a prudent reserve to handle any unforeseen event with a few extra dollars to boot. Instinctively, I believed that to achieve my goal to become a millionaire, I would need to make money from both my earned wages, along with select investments. One of the companies I was following closely was in the movie rental industry. The company had a vast library of movie selections to rent, all offered at a great price for consumers. There was plenty of opportunity in the entertainment space, and the video rental business was growing rapidly. I decided to take a bold step and buy stock warrants; each warrant was levered 10-fold. Each warrant holder had rights to buy a share of stock at a fixed price, for a period certain, in my case 18 months. If the stock price increased by 100%, I would make about 10 times my investment; if the stock price dropped by 10% or more, I would be likely to lose it all. This type of investing is called speculation. I knew the risks and considered that at my age, I could handle the loss. My luck paid off. The stock more than doubled and I cashed out of my $12,800 investment for $128,000. I was excited and relieved at the same time. Making the money is half the work, the other half is keeping it. In five years, I had seen peaks and troughs working as a broker. During this span, the market had crashed in 1987 and the Gulf War began in 1990. I knew this windfall was important, and I was not about to mismanage it.

$100,000 is a pretty good chunk of money when you've made it all from scratch. Immediately, a hundred-grand invested, if earning 7% a year, generates about $583 per month, by reinvesting the proceeds grows to $140,000 in five years. At that same 7% rate, the $140,000 generates $818 a month. The compounding effect is profound. After thorough consideration, I decided to diversify the $128,000 over several asset classes: stocks, bonds, cash, and real estate. My primary objective was to preserve my principle, increase my income, and grow my asset base. There is no perfect formula to investing. To succeed, it is necessary to remain adaptive to each person's individual circumstances and the economic whims dealt in the marketplace. For example, for young people the cost of raising a family is full of ongoing expenses. The outlays begin with autos, housing, diapers, childcare, health insurance, taxes, et cetera, and last through college. The list is endless and tough to manage. I knew that if I invested responsibly, my portfolio would work for me. I had two goals: 1) to financially provide for my family, and 2) to continue to build my net worth. The most important rule to investing is, "Do not lose money!" Stocks go down every day; how then is it possible not to lose money every now and then? If you have $100,000 invested in stocks, bonds, cash, and real estate, and the S&P 500 declines, the other investments can be in a position to cushion the fall. And what's promising, with history as our guide, the S&P 500 has been resilient.

Investor #3: Amassing $1,000,000

Whoever says that a million dollars' liquid is not very much anymore either has more money than they should, or has no idea what they are talking about. A million-dollar nest egg can grow significantly. A million dollar investment earning 5% generates $50,000 a year. I made my first investment score in 1990, and my second came in 1999. The internet was changing the landscape of American business virtually overnight. I had founded a discount brokerage firm and we were one of the early players to trade stocks online. During the internet craze, Yahoo was the leading search engine. Yahoo listed all companies in its search results numerically to alphabetically. Our company, 1DB.com, was the very first listing on Yahoo online search. It was a windfall for our small company. D.H. Blair, an old line Wall Street investment bank, offered to take our company public, which I initially accepted, and later rescinded as market conditions deteriorated when the tech bubble burst. It was at this stage my liquid net worth eclipsed the one-million-dollar mark.

Business Insider reports that it takes 32 years on average to accumulate one million dollars. This puts the group of self-made millionaires in the middle-aged category. Millionaires are usually very good at managing their expenses. Most millionaires are self-made and they know how difficult the journey has been to make the money and hold on to it. There are investment opportunities available only to millionaires classified as accredited investors. These high-net-worth investors can invest into hedge funds, private placements, partnerships, start-ups, rental properties, precious metals, options, and derivatives. This select group has accumulated sufficient assets enabling them to speculate with a portion of their capital on investments that offer higher return possibilities, if they choose. Millionaires are in rare air; they are in a position to have numerous investments working for them in concert. Just because they are in a position to take more risk doesn't mean these millionaires will do it. Millionaires are more often than not conservative investors. They do not want to lose their hard earned money. The equation to financial success is "earn more money than you spend." Self-made millionaires have this figured out.

They understand that if their capital is invested wisely, their portfolio grows prosperously.

Here is my suggestion for the typical middle aged baby boomer million-dollar portfolio:

Rule #1: *Do not <u>lose</u> money.*
Rule #2: *Never <u>forget</u> rule #1.*
Rule #3: *Buy the <u>best</u>.*

If you are looking to acquire the most valuable real estate, or purchase a legendary sports car, or earn a degree from the most elite university, you may want to consider Park Avenue in New York, a Ferrari, and Harvard University, respectively. Some might even say that each of these is the cream of the crop. What makes investing so amazing is that it doesn't take a ransom or a degree from an Ivy League institution to afford the best companies in the world. Most great companies are publicly owned and can be bought and sold as shares at reasonable price points. These best of the best companies are democratized, meaning that anyone can own them. Millionaires can afford to buy the very best and they never have to compromise on quality. They have learned that it is better to buy quality over the long haul. Rule #3 advocates only buying the best. Everything Warren Buffett owns in his portfolio is high quality. For millionaires to preserve and perpetuate their wealth, buying the best is a tried and true formula. There are countless investment strategies available to would-be financial gurus. I am a skeptic when it comes to these exotic methods and see these choices failing rule #3. Once again, buy the best. Many own the S&P 500 with its blue chip stocks for appreciation and its consistent dividends for income.

Choosing the right mixture of stocks and bonds depends on each person's particular situation. It also depends on the market's valuation. Logically, an investor would be more apt to increase their exposure to stocks when the valuation is at a discount to historical norms, and a lesser amount when the market is at a premium. Historically, the May through October period has been the weakest time to own stocks; some investors prefer decreasing or reallocating a portion of their stock holdings during these months, and again re-upping their stock holdings in the seasonally strong months of November through April. Preservation of capital, as well as maintaining purchasing power caused by inflation, is vitally important for middle-aged folks. Bonds are a key solution to solving this issue. Millionaires might consider purchasing investment grade tax-free municipals, taxable municipals, and intermediate to long-term corporate bonds, and ladder maturities from 2 to 15 years. When the 2-year bond matures or expires, they may replace it with a 15-year bond. As of this writing, the Federal Reserve is raising interest rates. If rates normalize in the next year or so, purchasing bonds that mature in 20 to 30 years is not out of the question. Treasury Inflation-Protected Securities are a secure investment and act as a hedge against rising consumer prices.

These instruments offer a nominal interest rate, with the principal increasing or decreasing with inflation and deflation.

Cash at times is king. Affluent investor portfolios can be well served with adequate amounts of cash for safety, opportunity, and unexpected surprises. Blue chip stocks and investment grade bonds are where I choose to invest the bulk of my assets and what I'd like to call my "main course." For appetizers, I tinker in small business interests (service providers), real estate investment trusts, gold, energy infrastructure-MLPs, S&P sectors, select growth stocks, share buy-backs, consumer services, IPOs, and federal budget targeted industries. For dessert, at times I sprinkle in a bit of speculation, such as trading call and put options for market timing situations (particularly after market pull-backs and corrections). Several of my favorite investment books are Ben Graham's classic, *The Intelligent Investor,* Sam Stovall's *Seven Rules of Wall Street,* John Bogle's *Common Sense Investing,* and Ray Dalio's *Principles: Life and Work.*

CHAPTER 7:

Nutrition: I Am What I Eat.

"Let food by thy medicine and medicine be thy food."
—Hippocrates

As a Tennessee boy growing up in the South, my knowledge of optimal nutrition was close to nil. My diet consisted of the following for breakfast: eggs, bacon, toast with butter and jelly, milk, cereal, French toast, country ham, biscuits and gravy, grits, hash browns, and oatmeal. Lunch consisted of sandwiches, lots of any kind of chips, burgers, hot dogs, and plenty of Coca-Cola. For dinner my mother would cook the best southern food around: fried okra, fried squash, mashed potatoes, scalloped potatoes, greens, casseroles, corn bread, pork chops, pot roast, and fried chicken, all washed down with homemade sweet tea. For dessert, I would feast on an abundance of sugar, ranging from pecan pie, brownies, chocolate chip cookies, chocolate oatmeal cookies, pound cake smothered in butter, to coconut cream pie. The food was always prepared and served with an abundance of love. Where I grew up, Southerners typically ate four meals a day, but only mentioned breakfast, lunch, and supper. The final meal was the traditional late-night snack. It entailed raiding the refrigerator or devouring one of my dad's fried bologna sandwiches with Louisiana hot sauce. The food was filling, tasty, and mostly cooked in a frying pan or on the grill. As for grilling and smoking up spare ribs and barbecue, Tennesseans are the best in the game.

I can attest that when it is time to eat in Clarksville, Tennessee, no food ever goes to waste; unfortunately, it does in time show up on our waistlines. It is not uncommon to see Southern folks dealing with the battle of the bulge—the food is too darn tasty. My journey from being a carefree, irresponsible, mischievous kid with a limited attention span, to a Wall Street desk jockey, to a marathoner (and later an ironman and ultra-runner) was nothing short of a modern-day miracle in my opinion. I had no discipline whatsoever when it came to what I ate or how much. All through growing up, and early in my career, I ate whatever I wanted and was oblivious to the health ramifications.

With increased training and competitions, my eating habits had to change—consuming excess sugar and unhealthy fats were dragging me down. No longer were the days of binging on fried chicken and Oreo cookies with ice cold milk the norm. Once I became immersed in my yoga journey, I consciously began to adapt my eating habits. I became aware of the connection between what I ate, and my performance and subsequent recovery. For instance, if I ate a Carvel sundae the evening prior to a 7 a.m. yoga class, I often felt sluggish and lethargic during my class. The same held true when it came to running. Bingeing on Fritos and freshly baked chocolate chip cookies on a Saturday night made me feel hungover during my early Sunday morning long run.

My athletic friend Dr. Donchey suggested the way for me to transform my eating habits was to give up meat, thus began my introduction to vegetarianism. This much I knew was true: between yoga and running, I needed a better mixture of fuel not only to survive the workouts, but to improve my fitness level. For me, the vegetarian diet consisted of the following carbohydrate-rich menu: pasta, pizza, rice, beans, bread, peanut butter, iceberg lettuce, Fluff, fruit smoothies with tons of fruit—especially bananas—and vegan protein.

On most nights, pasta filled me up, and I topped off my dinner with plenty of bread and butter. I was completely stuffed after every meal. Once I finished eating dinner, I often finished up any work I had outstanding and then I watched the news on TV. It never took long before I had my evening contemplation of whether or not I should eat a couple of freshly baked chocolate chip cookies. I was prone to purchasing Pillsbury cookie dough if by chance I found myself in the mood. This internal dialogue was repeated frequently. Should I have freshly baked cookies with milk or not? Rationalization would eventually win over any objections that might come to mind, such as, if you keep eating these cookies, you are going to gain weight. My internal rebuttal to this argument was that I only ate the cookies on a seldom basis. The truth was that I replayed this scenario almost on a daily basis with the cookies winning.

For the weekend, it was vegetarian a la carte, and that habitually meant pizza with double cheese extra cooked, sprinkled with parmesan cheese, chased with an IBC root beer (preferably with a frozen mug out of the freezer). I was genuinely motivated to live a healthier lifestyle, but I had limited knowledge when it came to proper nourishment. I was faithful to this menu for some time and often felt flat and hungry at odd hours of the day and night, which led to bingeing on peanut butter and marshmallow cream sandwiches.

Over the years, for obvious reasons, I didn't note much improvement—to either my waistline or my athletic performance. My menu was lacking, although it took me quite some time to figure out how or why. Getting one's nutrition right is a process: what works for one person, may not work for the next. To complicate matters, a diet that worked for me at one point may prove ineffective later. The more I learned to listen to my body, the more I began to tweak my eating habits based on what my body craved—beyond chocolate chip cookies!

As my athletic endeavors advanced and I spent more time training on a daily basis, I found it necessary to improve the quality of what I was putting into my body. A diet based on carbohydrates was draining me more often than not. My old, unhealthy eating habits, a la ice cream and cookies, still showed up on a weekly basis, but I was slowly and steadily shifting to healthier habits. Over time, by way of experimenting, I learned that eating whole foods—i.e., unprocessed food that is free from additives and artificial substances—had a positive impact my mental, emotional, and physical well-being. The more I ate whole foods, the more my body began demanding densely nutritious foods of the low-glycemic, or low-carb, sort. My staples became and remain the following: spinach, kale, collards, broccoli, red peppers, avocados, nuts, seeds, carrots, cauliflower, cucumbers, and limited amounts of fruits and berries. Highly nutritious vegetables are the glue that holds it all together for me. I have since added meat products back into my diet on a supplemental basis.

How do I feel at this point in my life after a dozen years of experimenting? It depends on the day; some days I feel great, other days I feel off or sluggish. For me, eating is just one part of how my body feels and responds. There are a number of factors that come into play, which include stress, genetics, sleep patterns, and the intensity of workout schedules. Nowadays, if I train and exercise for extensive periods of time, I will sometimes use carbohydrates to supplement my performance. I have learned that there is no one-size-fits-all, and adapting to ever-changing situations is the key to success when it comes to fueling for performance and health.

I believe food is to be consumed for its wholesomeness, vitality, and enjoyment. "All things in moderation" was an expression I heard often growing up in the South. Funny, I never knew what it meant. Why? Because moderation was not part of my life. I had two gears: on and off. I worked, played, and ate with abandon early on. When I was having fun, I would go until I dropped. If I was hungry or starving, I would eat like a horse. The principle of moderation, doing or consuming less over an extended period, never made sense to me until later in life. Today, I still like going for it, but I see moderation as an immutable truth to a healthy and fruitful existence.

Fountain of Youth

The question I'm asked most often is, "What does your diet entail?" In the previous paragraphs I provided an overview of where I came from health-wise and where I am today, and what I ate then versus what I eat now. We live in an information overload world, full of media blitz and sensationalism; it seems that just about everywhere there's a charlatan hawking the next miracle vitamin, herb, pill, or diet to instantly transform us. Many, if not most, of these purported life-changing solutions are farfetched. Athletes, movie stars, models, and the like are all targeted towards a "quick fix." According to the website HealthResearchFunding.org, 11% of male high school athletes have experimented with steroids. Using anabolic steroids can shorten a person's lifespan by years, and yet their usage is high behind closed doors. Far too often, we hear stories about people exceeding their limits by using performance-enhancing drugs; in short, they are putting their health at risk for immediate gratification. Unfortunately, people of all kinds can be, and at times are, seduced into spending money on these touted miracle substances. The truth is that there is no shortcut to healthy living; we must work at it.

Wellness is a lifestyle that comes from healthy living—eating nutritious food and partaking in strenuous exercise regularly. We spend our lives going to school, working, planning for our future, seeking our dream job, and ardently focusing on making money. Money, they say, makes the world go around. I beg to differ; I believe it takes a healthy body, mind, and spirit to make the world go around. Being physically fit is in my opinion, the "Fountain of Youth." Well-being is a mixture of mental, spiritual, and physical conditioning. It takes commitment and faith in oneself to become well-rounded in each of these areas. Wellness is a way of life that is contagious. When it comes to fitness, what works for some may not work for others; everyone has to find their own way, as in life. My spouse, Rosa, and our eldest daughter, Ashleigh, have made dance their core exercise discipline throughout their lives. The art of dancing is mentally stimulating and physically demanding. It's an excellent way to stay fit. While my son-in-law, Alex, prefers lifting weights. The point is that everyone is different and has his or her own interests.

By keeping our bodies in optimal condition, we can live out our dreams and play out our bucket list. I am a living example: over the past 10 years I've transformed myself health wise. I have more energy to accomplish my needs, wants, and goals today than I had five, ten, and fifteen years ago. And I am not alone—Americans are living longer. Breakthroughs in medical science have extended the lifespan of those blessed to be living in the developed world. I am 55 years old; according to the Social Security Administration's life expectancy calculator, I am expected to live until I am 82.8 years old; a female my age is now estimated to live to 85.9. In 1991, life expectancy for men and women was 72 and 78.9 years respectively; in 1916, it was 49.6 years for men and 54.3 years for women. Living a longer life is wonderful in every way, as long we are healthy and fit enough to enjoy ourselves each day. Research confirms that the more physically fit men and women keep themselves, the lower their chances of developing serious health conditions.

If physical fitness is the fountain of youth, then eating fresh wholesome food is the fuel that makes the fountain flow. As I said earlier, learning what to eat and when is a process. What works for some, won't work for all. In my case, I attribute a significant amount of my vitality and aptitude to what I call the "Green Drink." I've been drinking the Green Drink for three years now, and it has transformed me in the following ways: 1) My recovery time from long demanding workouts has been virtually cut in half; 2) I have energy throughout the day comparable to when I was in my 20s; 3) I rarely become sick and I constantly tax my body to the max; 4) The Green Drink is clean burning fuel, which means I don't experience the highs and lows that come from eating the wrong foods; and 5) It gives me a pickup instantly every time I drink it.

The Green Drink is high octane. It is full of essential vitamins, minerals, and nutrients that our body's need for optimal performance. I have found it to be the most powerful concoction there is. Why am I so sure? Because I am a living, breathing example of its power, and I know that the drink is chock full of the most nutrient dense foods on the planet. I found eating sufficient amounts of nutrient-rich foods to be challenging. When I ate large amounts of green leafy or cruciferous vegetables, my stomach felt bloated. After a few days, I had to cut back to feel normal again. One day while I was shopping at Whole Foods, I spoke with a knowledgeable employee in the produce section. He introduced me to the ANDI Guide. ANDI stands for the *aggregate nutrient density index* and it rates foods based on their nutrient content. Then and there, I stepped up my game. I finally learned which vegetables were the healthiest for me. Up to this point, I often drank fruit smoothies and loved the taste of them and the sugar rush as well. However, not only did I find myself hungry again in short order, I was adding weight on my body in the wrong places. It was then I switched to making veggie drinks. Instantly, I noticed that even though I was ingesting large volumes of vegetables, I was no longer feeling the effects of bloating. The Green Drink was working for me.

From the moment I finished drinking my first blender full of nutrient dense veggies, I felt a noticeable boost. I never realized that I was nutritionally deficient, yet, I was. In the months to follow, I began experimenting with assorted foods to test my body's reaction to various mixed vegetable combinations. During this period I perfected the Green Drink. So, if you are interested in a life-changing food source and want to take my word for it, here it is.

The Green Drink

- Start with a powerful blender; I use a Vitamix.
- The Green Drink ingredients are as follows: ample amounts of <u>collards</u>, <u>kale</u>, and/or <u>spinach</u>; broccoli, ginger, celery, carrots, basil, cauliflower, garlic and red peppers; sparse amounts of either strawberries, blackberries, raspberries, or blueberries; mixed nuts; mixed seeds; and I always add avocado with its hard <u>seed</u> (70% of the nutrients and fiber are in the seed); add in protein mix if you like for muscle recovery and taste benefits.

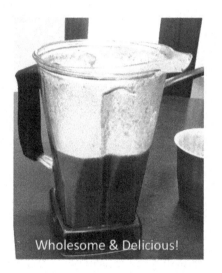
Wholesome & Delicious!

- For the liquid base, I use almond milk, water or coconut water, with plenty of ice.
- For athletes looking for even more of a punch, add maca powder, chia seeds, ginger, and turmeric root.
- This formula can transform your health. It is full of phytochemicals, antioxidants, essential vitamins, and minerals.

Tips for a longer, healthy life:

- Drink more water: women and men should drink 2 to 3 liters of water each day, respectively.

- Fast 12 hours: if your last meal or snack is at 10 p.m., wait until after 10 a.m. to eat anything else. Fasting for 12 hour intervals has scientific weight loss benefits (16 hour fasts are even better).

- Enjoy the sunshine: spend at least 15 minutes in the sun each day for your Vitamin D intake. Sunlight builds our immune systems, increases oxygen in the blood, wards off depression, lowers cholesterol, and kills harmful bacteria.

- Live to 100: eat whole foods, exercise daily, sleep 8 hours, consume moderately, and smile often!

- Last but not least: According to acclaimed cardiologist Dr. John Day, M.D., author of *The Longevity Plan*, smiling can add 7 years to your life. So, keep on smiling!

The Essence of Financial Fitness

"Most people don't plan to fail, they fail to plan."
-John D. MacArthur (Philanthropist)

As a veteran in the world of personal finance and financial planning, I am convinced that no two people are alike. What works for one personality type fails miserably for another. Some individuals are more cautious than others. A skydiver or mountain climber may see the world differently than a person who finds their thrill in bird watching or attending the opera. No matter how you slice it, people are distinct. Each of us has our own needs, wants, and priorities, and as we age, these attributes are constantly evolving. Personal financial planning is a dynamic process that changes throughout our life cycle. The key to making it all work is setting goals and objectives at each stage of your life, then mapping them out. In this lesson, I'm going to summarize five steps to achieving one's financial dreams and realizing one's goals.

Step One — Get Organized

Getting organized is easier than you think. The reason that so many people are in bad shape financially is because they see no way out of their predicament. Circumstances, environment, and behaviors are frequently cited as reasons why a person's financial status is in dire straits. I think most would agree that the only constant in life is change. If habits, situations, and developments are the explanations that describe our state of affairs, and at the same time everything is constantly changing, can't we change too? I believe that we can! The first step to financial fitness is getting organized.

Whether you are just starting out or have accumulated a large sum, Step One is the same for everyone. Organization is key! As a rule, I try to follow the principle that there's a place for everything, and everything in its place. Being organized isn't challenging; it is really pretty easy when you think about it. What is complicated and difficult is being disorganized. Financial failure is a bi-product of disarray and disorder. The good news is that Step One is a sure-fire way of getting on the right path. There are many ways to begin putting our affairs in order, just know that the state of being organized is ongoing. When it comes to mastering our personal finances the process isn't overly difficult, but does take some time.

A personal financial statement is the document used for organizing one's finances. A financial statement shows us what we own, what we owe, and our net worth. To create a financial statement I recommend using a spreadsheet, or online personal finance solution. I use Excel. There are templates on the web that make the process straightforward if you want to do it yourself, or you can employ the services of an accountant or a financial planner. To begin the process and get things underway, I believe in keeping things simple by creating a list using pen and paper. On your sheet of paper, draw a line down the middle. Label the left side "Assets" and the right side "Liabilities." List each of your assets by approximate monetary value: cash, cars, collectibles, clothes, jewelry, and anything that you can think of that you own that is worth something. On the other side of the sheet, write down your debts: credit cards, school loans, car loans, mortgages, and any outstanding obligations that you can think of no matter the size. Next, input each asset and each liability into the spreadsheet or personal finance application. Below is a sample of a personal financial statement.

Personal Financial Statement

Personal Financial Statement as of: _____ 12/31/2017 _____

Mrs. Networth	38
Name of Individual	Age

Mr. Networth	45
Spouse's Name	Age

1060 W Addison St, Chicago, IL 60613	Astronauts
Residence Address	Occupation

Assets		Liabilities	
1. Cash on hand and in Banks	$ 50,000	1. Accounts Payable	$ 7,500
2. Savings Accounts	$ 10,000	2. Notes Payable to Bank/Others (section 2)	$ 10,000
3. 401k, IRA Retirement Accounts	$ 140,000	3. Installment Account (Auto)	$
		Monthly Payment $	
4. Life Insurance – Cash Surrender Value)	$	4. Installment Accounts (Other)	$
5. Stocks and Bonds	$ 20,000	5. Loan on Life Insurance	$
6. Real Estate	$ 125,000	6. Mortgages on Real Estate (Section 4)	$ 100,000
7. Automobile – Present Value	$	7. Unpaid Taxes	$
8. Other Personal Property (Section 5)	$	8. Other Liabilities	$
9. Other Assets	$	Total Liabilities	$ 117,500
Total Assets	$ 345,000	9. Net Worth (Assets –Liabilities)	$ 227,500
		Total (Net Worth + Liabilities)	$ 345,000
		(this number should match total assets column)	
Section 1. Source of Income		**Contingent Liabilities**	
Salary	$ 75,000	As Endorser or Co-maker	$
Net Investment Income	$ 4,000	Legal Claims & Judgments	$
Real Estate Income	$ 10,000	Provisions for Income Taxes	$
Other Income (describe below)	$	Other Special Debt	$
Description of Other Income in Section 1			

Throughout my career, I have talked intimately with many millionaires, most whose net worth is between one to ten million dollars. Just about every one of these individuals had a sheet of paper or a printed spreadsheet that summarized their net worth. Even though it is simple, this sheet of paper is your personal financial statement. I will touch on this in more detail later in the book, but for now, let's keep things moving. After finishing up Step One, we are ready to move on to Step Two.

Step Two — Set Goals

Dream large. Think big. Go for it! According to the website Statistic Brain, approximately 45% of Americans make New Year's resolutions, and only 8% achieve them. Two things standout to me: over half the population doesn't even try making a resolution, and of those who do, the failure rate is a preposterous 92%. Here's a question—what's harder: saving five hundred dollars or losing five pounds? Both of these objectives are in most people's realm of possibilities. The first step to saving five hundred dollars is simple enough: earn money and set aside a portion each week until the target is met. The methodology is the same to accumulate a million dollars, only the numbers are larger. Who can lose five pounds? I think most people would agree that they could. Nutrition, athletics, and business success each involve accomplishing attainable goals. The easier the goal, the more realistic it will be to achieve it. I believe that writing down one's goals is essential. Let me say that again, if you want to achieve your goals, write them down! If my goal is to save $10 a day, after an extended period of meeting that goal, I can most likely raise the bar to $11, $12, or even $15. In a year's time, that adds up to $4,000. For those with larger purses, the same strategy applies, but the sums invested are larger. Set a saving goal and watch how fast it adds up.

In order to set proper goals, it is important to understand the reasons or the desires that move us toward attaining them. Our basic needs in the developed world start with money, food, shelter, clothing, healthcare, utilities, and fuel. There is no getting around the basics; we either address these needs tactically and methodically, or we suffer the consequences. If, for example, we need reliable transportation to travel back and forth from work to earn enough money to save for the future, the vehicle itself is very much an essential need. Let's say someone identifies a job or career they are passionate about, but it requires a college degree or a technical certification to obtain employment. The road to attaining the credentials necessary to be suitable for the position has become a basic need.

Funding these never-ending daily essentials is expensive. The cost of living itself is unrelenting. Many times I've been asked, "What drives me to make money?" The answer has always been the same: it costs a lot just to keep up with the daily expenses, and when I retire I want to have enough money so that I won't have to work. I may continue to work later in life, but it will be because I enjoy what I am doing, rather than out of necessity. I want to be able to live my golden years to the fullest. I have had to work hard for everything I've obtained. The key to all this is setting realistic, attainable goals. My ambition is to be able to retire with an annual income that I can live on without having to spend my savings and investments. I aim to live off the income, interest, dividends, and social security without depleting my accumulated principal. I came to realize that the only way I was going to attain the life I wanted was by making it happen. I would do this by setting definitive goals with specific timelines to completion.

My objective was to save ten percent of all my earnings on a weekly basis. As my bank account grew, I upped the ante, and in a couple of years my goals far outgrew my needs. 25 years later, I still practice these principles in all of my financial endeavors. The first part of my earnings goes into my traditional 401k retirement account. Why my retirement account? Several reasons: one, the tax write-off each year; two, the tax deferred growth; three, the assets may be exempt from the legal process. This means that no matter what happens along the way, these assets are inaccessible to creditors or unexpected lawsuits.

I've found setting goals in every area of my life rewarding. Whether I am trying to lose a few extra pounds, climb Mt. Whitney for the first time, participate as a volunteer for Junior Achievement, or write this book, it is all derived by my setting goals. I consider myself fortunate to have been born in America and raised by a family that loved me, who instilled me with humanitarian values and a strong work ethic. Those qualities enabled me to go out in the world and survive, but it has been my goals and aspirations that have taken me to the next level and enabled me to thrive.

Step Three — Map It Out

Mapping things out is one of my favorite pastimes. Mind mapping, or brainstorming, is the method I utilize to figure out what I want to accomplish and to prioritize. As a strategist and planner, I'm confounded that I have yet to see, hear, or even read about any financial services companies that offer brainstorming as part their client's comprehensive overview. Brainstorming or mind

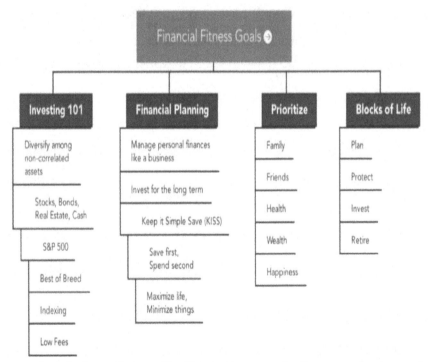

mapping is how I compile lists of my aspirations, projects, and dreams. I use Mindmeister.com as the cloud based software solution to put this into motion. Mindmeister is an easy to use application that organizes ideas and goals in a visual format. I learn best using a multisensory approach: a combination of pictures, diagrams, and words are what make things click for me. Brainstorming maps can be simple or complex, small in scope or unabridged, and if these working documents are stored in the cloud, they are always accessible. Each reference point (node) in the map can be linked to just about anything in the digital universe. Another great feature is that individual nodes are unrestricted, meaning they can be both a part of the initial mind map, and/or they can also be set up to be their own mind maps, as a map within a map. I know it's hard to visualize without using the application yourself, but I can tell you firsthand, it works well! When I work with others in a strategic planning or mind mapping session, I learn more about them than I ever would otherwise. In turn, I believe that all participants also learn something new about themselves.

I am convinced that whenever I change, the world as I see it changes. Working with a psychologist, I've found the best way for me to evolve and change is through self-examination. Philosopher Socrates said, "The unexamined life is not worth living." I believe that it takes self-awareness to accurately appraise oneself. Before I engage in   introspective analysis, I first try to examine my thinking, my actions, my reactions, and motives. Then I consider questions about where I am at this point, where I'd like to be, and how I am going to get there. I try to analyze each life goal from three different perspectives: 1) Why does this goal make sense for me? 2) What will it take for me to achieve it? 3) Did I grow as a person throughout the undertaking and attainment of this goal? I find that I achieve my goals much faster when I write them down.

Step Four — Adaptability

The only constant in life is change. No two days are alike. Whether we are working, going to school, training for a special event, or playing, each day contains its own nuances. I think that change can be either friend or foe, but one thing is certain: change is inevitable. I believe that to make change an ally we must be willing to accept it, remain flexible, and adapt accordingly. Step Four is more philosophical than technical in nature. I said there are five steps to achieving one's financial dreams. Every step serves a vital purpose, but Step Four is perhaps the most important of them all. Step Four is our reaction to situations, events, things, and people. There are those whose first reaction to something they find awkward or uncomfortable is flight or fight. If a teacher gives us a grade we don't deserve, or our boss is incompetent, or our coach is an egotist, our reaction to each of these people is significant. If we encounter a life-changing situation such as sickness, or get cheated out of our money or betrayed by someone, it is normal to get upset or angry. We must work to overcome these hardships and are often better in the end.

I learned early in my career that if someone stabs me in the back, I need to move on. I have been at this long enough to know that I no longer need to further my business relationships with misguided individuals. For me to move forward requires focusing on what is at hand. In order to achieve my dreams, I have to be looking ahead. My dreams and aspirations are in front of me, not behind. I'm sure that every reader has their own ideas and philosophy when it comes to dealing with change, so I will keep this section brief. The last thing I will say about change (good or bad), situations (good or bad), and people (good or bad) is that my reaction to each of these is what makes them so. Some people believe that all things happen for a reason. In that vein, alleged negatives or positives are experiences to learn and grow by. For me, the imperative is to be flexible with myself about whatever it is and adapt accordingly. I can seek the advice of others and choose the best options.

Step Five — Repetition

Repetition is the mother of success. Two birds named Pete and Repeat were sitting on a fence; Pete flew away, and who was left? Repeat. And the story goes on and on, infinitely. When I was a youngster, I found this riddle entertaining. Now, years later, I see repetition as a means to success. Einstein said, "The only source of knowledge is experience." It is my sense that humans are at their best in life's struggle. I'm not saying that it has to be a struggle to survive; I am saying that humans who thrive will most likely struggle. If you take a look at what makes us the proudest, it is most likely something that required enormous effort. For example, would I be more content winning the lottery or attaining financial success because of my effort and skill? Will I maximize my self-esteem by wasting time, or by learning something new that can evolve my life for the better? I'm not saying that there is anything wrong with leisure acts, but in my opinion the things that have helped me grow the most have required great effort in an ongoing manner.

We live in a fast paced world—arguably the fastest in history. New technologies via robots, augmented reality, artificial intelligence, and soon to be self-driving cars, are disrupting the way things have been done previously. This means that yesterday's skills will be less and less valuable in the world of tomorrow. How do we keep up or get ahead? We incorporate the abundant tools available to us to remain relevant. Social media has made the world much smaller and visible. A clever campaign that generates thousands of hits or likes can instantly bring anyone to the forefront. According to MarketingProfs, more than two million articles are published every day on the web. Classes are available online to learn just about anything for free or small sums via Massive Open Online Courses, known as MOOCs. You Tube statistics claim to have 300 hours of video added every minute. We are living in a new era; the digital age is a powerful locomotive. To rise to the top in today's world will require endless effort and networking. This is a good thing! I am not saying it is going to be easy, but I believe with commitment, discipline, and open-mindedness, a vast majority of enterprising individuals will succeed and shine beyond their imaginations.

I met a man in his late 70s at the gym early one Saturday morning. He was doing sit-ups—a lot of sit-ups. I could not take my eyes off this gent and found myself mesmerized by his output. He was doing sit-ups better than most fit 20-year-olds and far better than I ever had. When he finally stopped, I was stunned. I introduced myself to him and asked his age and how he was able to crush those sit-ups the way he did. He said without hesitation, "It just takes repetition."

In August 2015, I competed in the Leadville 100 race. This race is extraordinarily challenging because it starts at 10,000 feet elevation. Coming from Florida made this adventure one for the ages. Before the race, I met the race founder and legend, Ken Chlouber. Ken has a famous saying that exemplifies the benefits of showing up and repetition: "You're better than you think you are. You can do more than you think you can." I made it through that 100 miler, beat-up, exhausted, and cold. I was proud of myself. I have seen the benefits of repetition in every area of my life. Even today, I had a nutrient dense green drink for lunch and I'm going to yoga at 5 p.m.

CHAPTER 8:

Ironman Triathlon - Dealing with Adversity

"Dig deep into that inexhaustible
well of grit, guts, and determination."
—Ken Chlouber (Leadville 100)

It may sound strange, but I needed something new to keep my mind and body evolving. What's next syndrome was kicking in. Life has a way of knocking us down every once in a while. I had been dealing with a rough patch personally and professionally. As a 50-year-old, I'd grown to realize that everyone is subject to hardships at times in their life: poor health, financial setbacks, personal disasters, family crises, death, etc. For years, I'd perceived these occurrences to be unfortunate situations, what I called the alleged "bad things" in life. Now, as I look back, I am no longer sure if they were.

In many ways, these setbacks altered my internal compass for the better, and at times redirected the path of my life. The Great Recession of 2008 – 2009, also known as the housing crisis, hit the economy hard. 200,000 businesses closed during the recession and 9 million people lost their jobs. The banking and financial services industry—the field I worked in—was brought to its knees. The mid-size brokerage firm I ran felt like it was thrown into the middle of a multi-year hurricane. Stocks, housing, businesses, and interest rates fell into mega-bear market territory, which is defined as a drop of 40% or more. Individual 401(k) plans and IRA's were virtually cut in half. Our leaders in Washington fueled the flames by informing Americans that our country was on the cusp of a financial meltdown and economic depression. I'll express my opinion about all that at another time. As an investment professional managing money and leading a brokerage firm, the next five years were as tough as it gets.

The reality was, and is, that no one likes to lose money or their job, and both were happening. Fear was rampant, and with fear comes tightening up the belt, universally. Consumers immediately curtailed spending and increased their personal savings. In fact, personal savings escalated five-fold. Society went from saving less than 2% of their income to over 10%. The reason for the significant shift was fear. People were losing their jobs, equity in their homes and in their investment accounts, and they didn't know what economic calamity was coming next. For historical perspective, if you purchased blue chip stocks at the turn of the century (2000) and held them for ten straight years (2010), prices were down by 20%. In the investment community, this period is known as the lost decade. My mother used to always say, "When life gives you lemons, make lemonade." Every time she said that to me, it made me smile.

Running was my outlet through it all; it had become my escape hatch. No matter how difficult a given day, no matter the stress or drama, a run would change my state of mind. I found the more demanding the run, the greater the release from life's stressors. Wednesday night's track workout was the killer. I ran with the Wellington Runners Club and seldom missed a workout. Every week we would run different distances and paces. If we ran short distances, such as quarter-miles, it would feel like we were sprinting. If we ran half or full miles, the pace of the fast runners would torture the rest of us. I can't tell you how many times I showed up at the workout completely empty from the pressure I was living under. I would arrive and change out of my dress attire in my car in the parking lot. I had no idea how I was going to make it around that track, but I'd show up just the same. By 6:15 p.m. it was full on. My friends, the superstars, and I were laying it on the line out there. Invariably, my body responded and opened up. Every repetition was a test of my cardiovascular system and determination. I fed off the other runners who were working as hard as I was. One hour later, it was over. As I drove away in my car heading for home, I was a different person. It was like magic. Testing myself physically released my body from all of the tension and concerns that had held me captive.

After running the 113th and 114th Boston Marathons, I was ready for the next challenge. My fitness was at a level that led me to think I could tackle more. I continued participating in triathlons and had completed a couple of 70.3 mile, half-ironman triathlons. Running was my strongest discipline, with biking and swimming taking a back seat. There was something in me that was compelling me to keep moving forward. I decided I wanted to begin training for the full distance Ironman, totaling 140.6 miles. The Ironman is the capstone of the triathlon world. It consists of 2.4 miles ocean swimming, 112 miles biking, and 26.2 miles (a marathon) running, to finish it off. Undertaking the Ironman would require me to take my biking, swimming, and running, collectively, to the next dimension.

The inaugural New York Ironman Triathlon was scheduled for August 2012. I sat in front of my computer anxiously waiting to submit my application to participate. Ironman events typically sell out as quickly as sought-after rock concert tickets. As soon as Ironman opened the online process, I was on it. Initially, I didn't get accepted, but Ironman opened up additional entries at a higher price; I paid it. Concurrently, my best friend since our college days and medical mentor, Dr. Steven Donchey, was also accepted into the race. Two days later, while I was shopping at Whole Foods, I ran into Richard Wygand (nicknamed RW) at the checkout lane. RW is a local professional Ironman triathlete; I informed him of my acceptance into New York and asked him if he would coach me. He agreed. I had no idea how to train for an event of this magnitude and knew a coach would make all the difference. Twenty-four hours later, RW cranked up my training. I had a year to prepare for the race. I was in no rush whatsoever. I had learned that trying to achieve a certain fitness level too soon came with a cost—injury. I never suffered an acute injury that sidelined me for an extended period, but I had been affected by chronic problems in my feet, shins, and calves. Training with injuries is no fun, so this time I wanted to get there on my body's time frame.

RW suggested that I train for a half-ironman as an intermediate step to the full Ironman in New York; I agreed. The very next Saturday morning I began training with RW's triathlon group. These athletes welcomed me into the fold and made me feel part of the group right from the start. At the same time, these triathletes were hardcore. Every Saturday these guys would do what's called a BRIC workout. The workout consisted of two disciplines, both at full exertion. First, we'd ride 35 miles on the bike, and then immediately after, run 3 to 4 miles. At the onset of my Saturday rides with these thoroughbreds I would try to stay in the pace line with the group of riders for as long as I could, which typically meant until the halfway point. Then these guys would sprint up to 30 miles per hour on their bikes and leave me in the dust. I could not believe how fast they would ride. That would be the routine for months and months. I stayed with the group as long as I could and then they dropped me, which means I could not keep up with them any longer and was left behind. I finished half of those miles alone. Some of the rides would be 45 miles with longer runs afterwards. The pack would lose me at the halfway point and I'd struggle back on my own. Fast forward six months later, and I wasn't getting dropped anymore. My legs in the run after biking were springier, and my mind sharper. I was getting stronger. By the time the 70.3 event came around, I was ready. The conditions were tough: windy and rainy the first half of the race, and blistering hot the second half. I achieved the goal my coach and I wanted, and felt good about the result.

The Race - Ironman 140.6

Training for an Ironman and giving it one's best shot requires tremendous discipline and determination. To get into the proper shape, I trained between 15 to 17 hours weekly, spread out over six to seven days. I was swimming, running, and biking continuously. Every month the distances and tempo increased. Sundays were the long bike days. The long bike rides were mentally the most taxing part of the training. I had trained hard all week and then would be pushing on the bike 5 to 7 hours straight. This was pretty much the program up to the taper, two weeks before the race. After training for a year, it was time to race.

August 11, 2012, Steve and I woke up at 3:30 a.m. to catch one of the shuttle buses in Manhattan that would take the Ironman participants to the ferry. We met up with our friend, acclaimed equestrian Heather Caristo, and the three of us rode the ferry up the river to the race start. The current was ripping in our favor. This was a great boost for me as the ferry made its way to the starting line. I planned on racing this event buddying with my comrade-in-arms, Dr. Steve. We knew staying together during the race would act as a morale booster and allow us to share in the experience forever. That's not to say that we were going to hold anything back, quite the contrary.

Before I knew it, the waiting was over and I was diving into the Hudson River. Two days prior to the swim, two million gallons of sewage had spilled inadvertently into the river. Officials were so concerned that the swim was very close to being cancelled. The idea of swimming in the Hudson had me filled with trepidation, but there I was, giving it my all, competing in the New York City Ironman. I exited the water in 51 minutes, which was an incredibly fast time for me to swim 2.4 miles. As I hurried to the bike transition area, I looked for Steve. He was already preparing himself for the next 112 miles on the bike. It felt good to be on the bike. The course was mostly rolling hills and, coming from Florida a real test for me. I knew this was going to be a grind and it was. Mile after mile, hour after hour, I gritted it out. My bike had electronic shifters and with 11 miles remaining, the battery died. I was stuck in one gear. It was a high gear that required me to stand up out of the seat to keep the bike moving uphill. Fortunately, after a few miles it was mostly downhill or flat. I climbed off the bike in 6 hours, 45 minutes.

I had a marathon left to run, 26.2 miles. My legs were exhausted and felt like mush; Steve felt likewise. I had enough experience to know my legs would improve once I'd run a few miles. One by one, the miles went by. As I ran across the George Washington Bridge into Manhattan, I felt like I was accomplishing something special. It had nothing to do with anyone or anything; this was about me. As the sun fell and nightfall set in, it became difficult for me to see my steps. I stumbled a few times, but managed to steady myself. I could hear the spectators off in the distance, and knew I was getting closer and closer to the finish line. The last mile, I was full of joy. There were fans congratulating all the athletes and it felt really good. Steve and I crossed the finish line together. What an experience it was. The announcer over the loudspeaker said, "William Corley, you are an Ironman."

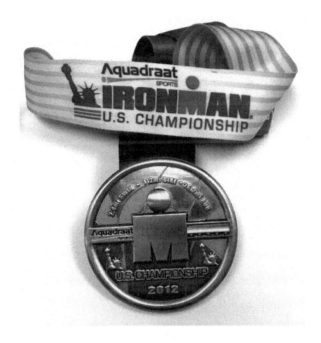

The Blocks of Life

"The world is like a grand staircase,
some are going up and some are going down."
— Samuel Johnson (Essayist)

Leonardo Da Vinci said, "Simplicity is the ultimate sophistication." Personally, I've noticed that just because something is simple in theory, doesn't mean it's easy in practice. For example, most people want the best for themselves and their families, such as a nice, safe place to live; reliable transportation, good schools, fun hobbies and recreation, the ability to provide the best for their children and pets; and to have sufficient savings for their retirement. To plan for each of these can be simple enough, but executing the plan isn't always so easy. For me to execute a plan effectively, it needs to be carefully considered and plotted in an organized and well-documented manner. Here is a real life story to explain what I mean. I met with a young couple to discuss financial planning and their future in general. Both of them were young professionals: she was a lawyer and he was an engineer. They were smart, earnest people and wanted to make the best decisions for themselves and their daughter. Collectively, they had many questions, which I did my best to answer. During our meeting, both husband and wife were at odds on some points and in agreement with others. One question led to another and then another. After several hours, I suggested that we reconvene in a week's time to give them the chance to sort out their decision.

They agreed. At our follow up meeting, I reiterated the points of agreement to see if they still felt the same way; they did. Next, I opened the discussion around their previous differences and asked what they had come up with since our last visit. At this point they both smiled sheepishly and said, "We haven't come up with anything." When I asked them why, they told me they had talked about it a little, but got lost in the subject matter.

As a multisensory person, I find the more senses I can bring to a decision the better. When it comes to financial fitness the subject is vast, and it can be overwhelming. So, a number of years ago, I crafted from wooden square blocks what I call the *Blocks of Life.* There are words on each block that represent intangibles most find important. I use the *Blocks of Life* to better illustrate financial planning, and proceeded 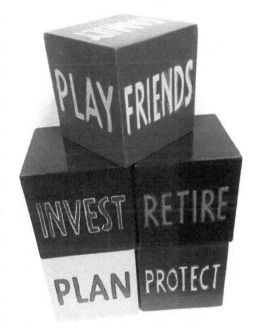 to share the basics noted below with this couple. The main block, *The Block of Life,* comprises those things most important to all of us: family, friends, health, wealth, and happiness. The next three blocks are colored in the manner of a traffic light and represent the essentials needed to succeed financially.

Financial fitness begins with the yellow block; it represents planning. When a traffic light is flashing yellow, it means to proceed with caution. The same applies to traveling the road to financial success. By reading this chapter and better acquainting yourself with personal finance, you are certainly proceeding with caution. The best way to drive through the yellow light is to slow down, check the mirrors, and look both ways. The yellow block serves as a reminder that to successfully navigate your journey, it is best to <u>plan</u>.

Next is the green block; it signifies investing. A green traffic light signals us to move forward. Not moving forward or going backwards at a green light would disrupt traffic for everyone. When it comes to one's finances, green is good. A green light indicates that wise decisions have been made. For most, that means they have a decent paying job, they are living within their means, and are making positive things happen in their lives. During this green-light period, individuals are saving and investing regularly, and building their net worth. From my viewpoint, anyone who reaches their own personal green light is on their way to financial success.

The red block signifies danger. It's what I consider our wake-up call block. When we reach this point, it's time to reassess, ask formative questions about where we are, and gain clarity on how we arrived at this point. Spotting warning signs and implementing strategies to ward off danger is vitally important to our prolonged success. If we ignore the warning signs, we are putting our financial fitness in jeopardy. Without proper planning and guidance, many people remain in the danger zone, which hurts them, both over the short and long term.

What are these potential dangers to which I am referring? Predatory lawsuits, sour business deals, bad investments, sicknesses or injuries, disability, and even death. Nobody expects these calamities will happen to them, but they do happen to people every day, and it is more often than you think. Additional dangers include rapacious attorneys and wallet-busting bankruptcies. To protect yourself over the course of your life from these pitfalls, you need to make sure that a large share of your financial holdings is in areas that are exempt from the legal process. In most states, retirement plans, home ownership, annuities and life insurance proceeds are non-attachable assets, which mean these assets are sheltered from harm's way. For more information about asset protection, I recommend consulting with a legal expert and a reputable financial planner to make certain your assets are directed accordingly.

One of the questions that I frequently ask new clients is, "What do you consider to be your most important financial asset?" They invariably answer with "my house, my investment portfolio, and my car." I've even heard "my dog." The single most valuable asset most of us possess is our ability to earn an income. What happens to our dreams if we are incapable of working because of disability? According to the Social Security Administration, 56 million Americans, or one in five, live with disabilities. It can happen to any of us. Accidents and illnesses can turn lives upside down; disabilities can prevent people from working and earning money. There is a solution: long-term disability insurance. Did you know that there are disability insurance policies that at retirement will refund you all your premiums, less any claims? For death protection, there is life insurance. Term insurance is what is mostly touted for life insurance buyers, yet in this period of zero interest rates with limited options for guaranteed safety, permanent life insurance is safe.

Our final block in the financial fitness story is the blue block. The blue block represents retirement, financial independence and hopefully, blue skies ahead. Ideally, at this juncture folks have protected themselves against the wiles of the world and have diligently saved and invested wisely. Much of the financial success at this stage is a product of self-reliance. By taking ownership and accountability for our futures we are more likely to make it. Financially fit folks learn they are responsible for taking care of themselves; at the same time, at least in my case, we welcome and appreciate any and all acts of kindness along the way.

This is the time in life when we see clearly the benefits of our decision making. By foregoing immediate gratification periodically, and investing those extra proceeds into our savings and retirement accounts, we put ourselves in a position to harvest the bounty of our efforts. By making smart decisions we are now in a position to reap the rewards. We've learned that things don't always go as planned, and we've witnessed episodes when financial markets went from bad to worse, testing our nerves, and losing us money. It was during these dark days that we had the fortitude to tighten our belts even more so, and stepped up our savings to help make up for the financial shortfall. Every dollar that we saved and invested over the years has been working for us. Those dollars invested have earned us interest, dividends, and hopefully appreciation in tandem with the growth of the economy. It's wonderful to see that those small sums of pennies and dollars invested over the years have now appreciated to large sums. Blue skies are awaiting all of us, as long as we save early and often.

CHAPTER 9:

D.N.F.

*"The greater danger for most lies not in aiming too high
and falling short, but in aiming too low and hitting our mark."*
—Michelangelo (Artist)

At this point, I had upped my game by completing a number of 50 kilometer and 50 mile running races, to include the grueling Destin 50 miler, which was run start to finish on the sand between the Destin Pass and Seagrove along the Gulf of Mexico. What had I learned? That it took continuous training, focus, and commitment to survive these races. I had watched friends enter and successfully complete 100 mile races for at least a year, marveling at their ability to stay with the torture for a full 100 miles. The thing was, I wasn't sure if I had it in me to complete 100 miles, but the more I conferred with ultra-running friends, the more I learned that no one was ever sure, and that no matter how much one had trained and planned, 100 miles was a long way to go and anything could go wrong, or for that matter, right, too.

When it comes to participating in endurance sports racing, there are three words that athletes most definitely do not want to hear: "Did Not Finish," better known by the acronym, D.N.F. It takes a fair amount of courage just to show up at the starting line of an ultramarathon, which is any distance greater than 26.2 miles. But when it comes to toeing the starting line for your first hundred-mile event, it's a tall order. Up to this point in my endurance racing career, I had completed every race that I competed in. In fact, the thought of not finishing was not an option. I had never won any of these events outright, but I had given each of the challenges my best effort and crossed the finish line.

Ever since I was a young boy, I put my all into whatever sports competition I was involved in. Whether that meant climbing a tree, racing on the playground, or competing in team sports or backyard games with my neighbors, I played to win. As I've said throughout this book, I wasn't prone to winning, but I tried my hardest just the same. When I was 12 years old, I was backup quarterback for my pee-wee football team, the Falcons. One game, when we were playing against the Packers—the best team in the league—our starting quarterback took a hit and became injured. That meant it was time for me, the replacement, to play. With only a few minutes to go in the game, I ran for a touchdown, and we ended up tying the Packers, which to me was like winning a championship. My Dad was my coach and afterwards gave me a trophy with the engraving, "He did not quit." As I have noted previously, I was a mediocre athlete at best, but my father encouraged me as if I were a star. Even then, I knew the trophy was more a show of my father's love for his son than a symbol of my athleticism, but it meant something to me just the same: if you try and give it your all, anything is possible.

The Grand Tetons 100, located in Northwestern Wyoming, was the race I selected for my inaugural 100 miles in October 2013. Wyoming is known for its mountains, fresh air, majestic beauty, snow skiing, hiking, rock climbing, and everything outdoors. The Grand Tetons offer pristine mountains, clear lakes, thick woodlands, and wild animals to boot, particularly bears. Coming from Florida, I knew the mountains would be a respite for my soul. I looked forward to magnificent vista views, breathing in the fresh mountain air, and running long and far in the cool temperatures of October. The setting of this race was completely different from South Florida's flatlands, heat, and humidity. The other appealing element of this race was that it was run on roads. Roads meant I would not have to navigate treacherous mountain trails. For my first attempt, that appealed to me. Also appealing were the facts that the race director was legendary ultra-marathoner Lisa Batchen (who is now my coach), and my friend and client Jodi Weiss (30 time 100-mile finisher) let me run and share crew with her. I was hopeful that I would be able to complete this ultramarathon and attain a 100-mile buckle. It is worth noting that for 100 mile races, buckles—as in belt buckles with the race name on it—are the equivalent of medals. Everyone who runs ultramarathons aspires to earn their first 100-mile buckle, and there's a cost, pain!

Everything they say about the beauty and majestic nature of the Grand Tetons is true. But it was cold. Really cold! In fact, it snowed the two days prior to the race. Coming from 80+ degrees, cold weather, let alone snow, was a shock. I had run plenty of races in undesirable weather conditions and uncomfortable temperatures, but never for more than a few hours. Finishing the Grand Tetons

100 ultramarathon would take me approximately 30 hours and surely test my mettle. As I waited for the race to get underway in the wee hours of morning, I was freezing. The outdoor thermometer read 20 degrees—not ideal for Florida runners. And just like that, we were off and running. I was bundled up with three layers and a coat—if a massive snowstorm was to hit, I was prepared, ski mittens and all. The conditions were such that by mile 10 my water bottle froze. I did not have water to drink until I met up with the support crew. My only wish as each mile passed was that it would warm up at some point. I was desperate to get into a groove and to forget the cold, but it persisted.

Running on the road was a positive. Every little positive counted. I didn't have to worry about getting lost, or tripping over a root or rock as I would on a trail. By the time I covered the first of nearly four marathon distances of 26.2 miles, I was feeling optimistic. My legs were managing the rolling mountain roads better than I had expected. The miles were happening. I passed 30, 35, 40, 45, and 50. Fifty miles was the farthest that I had ever ran. Everything was good, until it wasn't.

At mile 50, I began to feel the effects of the wear and tear on my body. The freezing temperatures had taken me by surprise, and it was getting colder again. I was so far out of my comfort zone that I was residing in what I'd call my personal no man's land. Whenever I needed to stop and relieve myself during this race (or any ultra-distance outing), I paid extra attention to the color of my urine to effectively manage my fluid intake. During my 50-mile check, I noticed the color of my urine was far from normal: it was red, indicating that I was bleeding internally. It scared me. I tried to be level headed, yet at the same time this had never happened to me before. Our crew and the race director were matter of fact: they asked how much I had been drinking, and explained that it was a function of my being dehydrated. Apparently, this was not an uncommon occurrence. Their response helped, but I was nervous. I decided then and there to call my pal, Dr. Donchey. Fortunately, I was able to reach him on his cell phone and I explained my health scare. He listened carefully to what I had to say and told me to keep a close eye on the situation and to let him know if it got any worse. With that, I pulled myself together and proceeded back to the highway picking up where I'd left off, with 50 miles left to go.

I had been at it for over 12 hours. Days are short in the Tetons, and as sunset neared, the weather worsened. Up to this point, temperatures had warmed up to the high 30s from daylight and the sun's rays. As the clock passed 6:00 p.m., the air resumed its frigid chill. The wind began blowing harder and the temperature dropped, and then it was night. During the next several hours it went from cold, to freezing cold; the temperature fell under 20 degrees Fahrenheit with 25 mile-per-hour sustained winds. I was trembling and my teeth were chattering. I felt like my body was on the cusp of hypothermia. I was no longer running, only walking, and my pace was slowing by the minute. I was becoming a drag and weak link to the others around me. My personal resolve had abandoned me. I felt desperate.

If you consciously pull yourself out of a race, it results in a D.N.F. It's throwing in the towel, raising the white flag; to me, it's an unconditional surrender, a loss. If I chose to quit I would be letting down my running mate, our crew, and myself. It would be a selfish choice of sorts. If I stopped, we all stopped, as the hotel was hours away. Everyone was prepared to keep moving forward, and they were waiting for me to make my decision. Will I keep going or not? I asked myself, "What will it be?" I was 62 miles into the race with 38 to go. It was the furthest I had ever run, and I had a full night and the following day's run remaining to obtain ultra-marathon preeminence.

The race director showed up precisely at my location as I was contemplating my fate, quitting. A tried and true ultra-legend, a master in the art of overcoming one's pain, Lisa offered her insights. She painted an optimistic picture, assuring me that others had been in the exact place I was in at that moment, and that I was more than capable of persisting to the end. My crew and running mate were leaving it up to me. Will this be my time, perhaps a once in a lifetime chance, to take my game to the next level? I was nearing my personal breaking point. I was over it. The cold was crushing my spirit. Could I find it in my gut to dig deep enough to rise to the occasion, or would this moment become my personal ultra-running Waterloo? The truth was that I felt distraught, disconnected, and disinterested, not to mention that I was frozen, sick, and tired. I was ready to take the D.N.F., get myself to a warm hotel where I could sleep it off, and hang up my 100-mile dreams, forever!

Beaten Not Broken

"Time solves ninety percent of all problems."
—Dr. William H. Corley (Theologian)

Ancient scriptures proclaim everything happens for a reason. I have pondered this ideology on and off for years, and I still do. In one vein it makes sense to me, in another, it does not. It is hard for me to wrap my mind around the darkness in society that breeds violent crime, hatred, starvation, child abuse, war, racism, self-righteous condemnation, uncivilized discourse, political polarity, elitism, and judgmentalism. I cannot understand how perpetrators of such selfish acts can live with themselves. I've grappled with the question why bad things happen to good people. And why is it that actions of the unjust are often borne upon those who are just. For me, the answer to these questions is a mystery, it remains unknowable.

Growing older and reflecting in the rear view mirror of my life, there seems to be a purpose playing itself out. It's as if there is a celestial guide of sorts pointing me in the right direction, and there are reasons for each segment of my life up to now. I've observed this in things such as friendships, unusual coincidences, serendipitous encounters, and life's close calls, even with complete strangers. I've witnessed these twists of fate in good times, bad times, and in countless situations. The more I examine these occurrences, the more intrigued I am about the possibility of divine purpose. How can this be? How can there be a preordained plan for humans possessed with free will? Are we not the captains of our ships? Don't we all make the decisions in our lives? Yes, we do. And, in scrutinizing those decisions, don't they appear to string themselves together in an orderly way of sorts? For example, if we do well in school, graduate college, get a good job, live in the right neighborhood, associate with the right people, exercise regularly, eat properly, treat others respectfully, and plan ahead, isn't life supposed to be swell? That's pretty much the way I thought it was meant to be. In this context, it looks obvious to me like we are the ones responsible for much of our outcomes. But then, when it is least expected, calamity strikes and order instantly gives way to disorder. What felt stable and secure becomes upended by uncertainty. The good fortune attained by playing the part of the good actor suddenly transforms into misfortune, and if things continue to fall apart, it can lead to chaos and possibly utter ruin. What happens then?

I'll tell you what I think happens. We get knocked down. It could be a family situation that punches us in the gut, or a financial calamity, a freak accident, a health crisis, even death. I was told by a very wise man that catastrophic situations hit everyone at multiple times in their lives. No one is exempt. So, how is this doom and gloom part of a higher intelligence? In my case, I am beginning to see all of these seeming failures and setbacks as life changing events that have altered the course of my life. Such formidable circumstances forced me into making completely different decisions to find my way, requiring me to let go of the past and be willing to accept what was in store for me at that moment. Am I really in charge of my life after all, or is destiny my lifelong partner?

My grandfather, "Fearless Ferns," was a professional welterweight boxer. When I was a boy, he used to say, "The bigger they are, the harder they fall." I never really understood what he meant at the time, but as I grew up, I grasped the meaning, both literally and figuratively. Literally, a large stature fighter that gets knocked to the floor hits the canvas like an oak tree with a loud thud. Figuratively, a 13-year old business, like my own that employs 50 plus people with thousands of customers, that falls on hard times also hits the canvas with a loud thud. The difference between the two is a business thud affects far more people, and the fallout, with punishing tremors and ripples, lasts far longer than imaginable.

In 2008, financial services firms, one after another, bit the dust. Home prices fell by 30% nationwide, stock prices sunk over 50%, job losses were at 700,000 per month, and companies, particularly in the financial space, were shuttering their doors like an epidemic. And there I was running a stock brokerage firm—a kid from Clarksville, Tennessee—certain to get washed away and drown in this perfect storm. Our firm and franchisees were hit from all sides. Financially we were no longer making a profit; in fact, we were generating outsized losses. Every day the stock market would continue its negative spiral. Customers that leveraged their accounts to make larger returns were getting margin calls to pay back the loans on a daily basis. Investors were more than disgruntled with their asset values dwindling and the country upside down from the great recession; plaintiff lawyers were waiting in the weeds to attack anywhere they could. In Washington, the political bourgeoisie were pointing fingers and casting blame on anybody but themselves; banks and brokerage houses became their primary targets. Let me say right here and now, our small company was absolutely in no way whatsoever part of the Wall Street apparatus. But when it all came crashing down, we were smack in the middle of the wake of the furor.

Our business was ambushed from all sides. I had built this company from the ground up day by day, year over year; now it was unraveling. There was no way I could hold it all together alone; I needed support. Fortunately, I got it. Aileen Gallagher is our firm's chief financial officer. Aileen has a razor sharp intellect and unparalleled reasoning skills, accompanied with steely nerves. No matter how bad things got, I could always count on Aileen. As CFO, Aileen knew our company's financial status at all times. She was my go to person before I made any important decision.

It seemed as if our company was in a black hole spiraling to its demise. Directions for every step the company took were imparted by our attorney and general counsel Robert G. Haile, Jr. Rob is the most skilled extemporaneous speaker I have ever witnessed; his litigation skills are unparalleled. The mass of predatory lawsuits, employee defections and regulatory compression frightened clientele; lying in wait for the next shoe to drop was paralyzing. We were battling in the trenches and fighting for our lives on a daily basis.

Since our inception working together, the executive team, consisting of Nicky Cheng (Chief Compliance Officer), Joel De Young (Chief Operating Officer), Aileen Gallagher (Chief Financial Officer), and me (Chief Executive Officer), operated the company on conservative principles and were frugal with the company's finances. We saved diligently during the good times and built a respectable balance sheet from the company's retained earnings. Until recently, we would only draw from the proceeds to grow the business or make acquisitions. Things were different now; a once thriving, profitable company was losing $200,000 per month. It was not so much the operation itself that was bleeding the company; it was more the externalities that came from the economic meltdown. Those were trying times that required digging in by the nails and holding on at all costs. Desperate times called for desperate measures. To survive meant that the company would have to be restructured, overhauled is more like it. Every item on the income statement had to be meticulously called into question. The company was now being run from the expense side, with all costs being examined for absolute necessity. Restructuring began with us curtailing the largest expenses first.

We moved to smaller offices, laid-off inessential workers, froze wages, renegotiated with our technology vendors, and just plain tightened our belts. Every month from then on we continued to cut any costs that we could. Legal expense, which was now the largest drain on the firm, was an area that we couldn't eliminate. Not only was I losing substantial amounts of money, for extended periods I wasn't even receiving my salary. I was working for free. This squeezing savings from wherever we could became the norm. I had no way of knowing how long this would last or what the outcome would be. The entire episode totaled eight years. It was the most difficult ordeal I ever experienced. Keeping the company afloat when the problems just continued to surface was beyond my scope. Somehow, with the core of our management team, we held it together. We stood shoulder-to-shoulder through it all; we were united in our purpose, and when it was all said and done, we made it.

This brings me back to the premise, "Everything happens for a reason." How could I have possibly benefitted from this grueling period? Am I glad it happened? No. Do I still wish the company had the money it lost? Yes, that's for sure, and it is a reason that I'm still hard at it, working away. Am I better off now emotionally, mentally, psychologically, then before? I don't know. What I do know is that I'm older, and as the years have piled on, the experiences have, too. So, what's the redeeming purpose in my life from all this? Did I grow as a person, or benefit in some manner? I think the answer to these questions is imperceptible, meaning it isn't black or white; the answer is not scientific. But in reflection, I see things evidence-based.

From the events surrounding this epic economic contraction, our business dramatically changed. To survive we had to do many things differently. Additionally, we as people, me in particular as the leader, had to adapt and change. These changes personally have made me a better version of myself to others, and have also brought me closer to my core. When the company was larger, I was subject to its whims. There was endless drama. I had managers to handle most of the noise, but the big problems always landed on my desk. It wasn't the job I preferred. I wanted to create better ways of investing. My mission was to make our clients' money. I wanted to be the very best at managing our clients' assets. As the company grew, my responsibilities and the time constraints associated with those obligations pulled me in other directions. It took turning things upside down for me to get back to my chief passion and what drives me still: making money in the financial markets.

Our company weathered the storm and has repositioned itself to once again succeed and thrive in this new age of investing. Am I happier now than before? As a person and leader, I am sturdier, more secure, and more confident in my decision making. I have gained wisdom from being tested under fire. The company's future is brighter from the changes we implemented. My competency has evolved to that of a financial strategist. I have spent 50 hours or more a week for a decade studying the investment markets and their histories. I have an unquenchable curiosity of how financial markets function under all economic backdrops, and which investments are most suitable for profitable gain during expansionary or contractionary periods. My expertise as a money manager and 30-year industry veteran is well tested. I believe that the best days of my life are in front of me. I feel that I am in a position to make not only my life more fulfilling, but to positively impact the lives of others financially. In comparison to before when the company was still flying high, I am having a lot more fun and I am happier today. For that, I am grateful for the way destiny has reshaped my life.

CHAPTER 10:

If at First You Don't Succeed...

*"The one who is constant in happiness
must frequently change."*
—Confucius

After my undesirable D.N.F. at the Grand Tetons 100-mile race in October, I was determined to get this setback behind me. Several experienced ultra-marathoners shared with me that there were two fates when it came down to erasing a failed 100-mile ultramarathon attempt: either I could wallow in it, or I could tackle it head-on and overcome it. There was no way I wanted a D.N.F. looming over me; I needed to attempt a 100-miler ASAP and cross the finish line.

I signed up for the Wild Sebastian 100 the next month. The race takes place in St. Sebastian River State Park, in Fellsmere, Florida. Coincidentally, the location was precisely 100 miles from my house (a good omen). With trepidation, but determination, I signed up and asked ultra-running veteran Jodi to pace me once again. She had completed Wild Sebastian 100 the prior year, so she knew her way around the course. After the Grand Tetons debacle, I let her know that I needed to complete the race for my psyche.

I knew what I must do to make completing this race a reality; I was going to have to push myself further than ever before. I would have to accept the pain, become one with it, and get over myself. When my feet ached and throbbed, as they surely would, I was going to have to keep going. When fatigue set in from staying awake and moving for so many hours, somehow, I would just have to manage. Thinking about it in the days leading up to the race was worrisome. I would be testing myself like never before, but I wanted to finish this 100-mile ultra. Jodi would set the pace, and my game plan was just to follow her lead and to hold on for dear life.

Four weeks later, the 2013 Wild Sebastian 100 was underway. Growing up in the hills of Tennessee, I was accustomed to getting dirty and grungy playing in red clay turf. The Wild Sebastian course was full of roots, rocks, some high grass and soil that seemed manageable to me, but to my dismay, this was not the case. The course was full of mucky pools of stagnant water, sugar sand, sand spurs, and hog ruts. At mile three in the race, I found the terrain unforgiving with me slogging my way through what looked like the swamp where Shrek lived. I was starting to regret my decision to attempt this 100-mile battle; I was at mile 5.

Thirty minutes later the situation began to improve. I finally exited Shrek's swamp and the terrain changed. After crossing through a fence, we ran in the middle of some remote field adjacent to I-95 in weeds waist high. The place was surreal. I could deal with the weeds though, because the lead runners were blazing a trail by stomping down the high grass; it was a pathway for those of us bringing up the rear. As we reached each aid station we were greeted by cheerful volunteers who readily assisted us with drinks, snacks and whatever we needed. Life was looking up

— I started to imagine I could manage this 100-mile ultra and possibly finish. But I had a long way to go: Wild Sebastian consisted of four twenty-five mile loops with at least half of those miles on highly technical terrain.

I've shared plenty of details pertaining to each of my races in the previous chapters: the misery, the dread, the pulling myself together and whatnot. To avoid being repetitive, I'm going to summarize how this 100 played out. The race course went from trail, to swamp, to weeds, to cypress stumps, to sugar sand, to vines, prickly plants, gnarly roots, pot holes, and ruts created from wild boar herds, and finally to nirvana — a three-mile stretch of dirt road. As 100-milers, we feasted on this banquet of terrain as a four-course adventure.

We ran through smelly black water. There were colorful snakes, not ones that you would ever wish to be bitten by. It was hot enough out to sweat at all times. We ran in quicksand, four times. We ran farther and farther and completed lap after lap, mile after mile. I decided that I needed a break at mile 75. It was after midnight, and I'd been at this for over 20 hours. I sat down in a chair at the aid station, and it was eternal bliss. I wanted to stay there for the rest of my life, but then General Jodi barked out the order, "You're wasting time; let's get moving." I was stricken by the horror of going back out on that final loop for another 25 miles. It seemed utterly barbaric to me. And that's what I was thinking as I moseyed back on the course and disappeared into the swamp in the pitch black hours of night.

We kept running and walking, breathing and talking. Those hours were dark times for me, literally and figuratively. Jodi's resolve was steely, unwavering. She'd say, "Just keep moving forward." There were episodes when we ran fast, which were followed by us having to calm it all down. That was our saying, "Calm it all down." Daylight came and with it optimistic thoughts. The new dawn was like a sign that this was not only possible, but that it was going to happen. With 15 miles to go two of my Ironman pals, Craig and Gary, surprised me by showing up on mountain bikes. They brought me a cold beer that I guzzled instantly. They were my final confirmation; I knew I was going to finish. It finally ended in 30 hours, 24 minutes and 52 seconds. I had completed my first hundred-miler, and I had a Wild Sebastion100 buckle to show for it, in addition to destroyed feet, and a repaired ego.

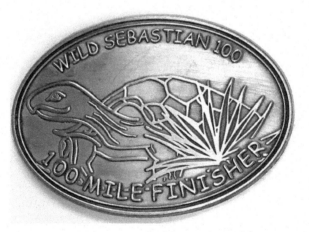

Quitters Can Win and Win Big!

"Winners never quit and quitters never win."

-*Vince Lombardi*

Lombardi's quote embodies an idyllic bravado of herculean proportion. To me, the quote is cliché at best, and when accompanied by the word "never," mostly inaccurate. I remember working at a major grocery store chain in my late teens as a customer-service attendant, better known as a bag boy. The job was demeaning. I disliked every minute that I spent working there. After only a few days of working, I crossed paths with an employee in the stocking department that had been working there for a couple of years. I vaguely knew him from high school, but contrary to his lowly social status at high school, at work he thought he was hot stuff. He would flaunt his higher wage around and abuse his seniority by belittling my position. Outside this grocery store chain, this guy was anti-cool. Even though I was a young man with limited life skills and virtually no experience at the time, the idea of this person ranking himself over me didn't sit right with me. I wouldn't call myself the coolest cat around growing up, but I can honestly say that I was no dork. My parents taught me to treat people of all races and walks of life with respect. This clown knew nothing about mutual respect, and on days our schedules coincided, I would intentionally avoid him. It didn't take me long to figure out that being a bag boy came with a considerable amount of hazing.

Fourth of July weekend is a national treasure. It's an uplifting holiday in the midst of summer and Americans are primed for fun, food, fireworks, and festivities. In order to prep for the 4th, folks visit their local supermarket to load up with all the best eats and drinks. Days leading up to the holiday, the store was bursting at the seams with every checkout lane full of high-spirited soon-to-be celebrators. As a grocery store employee, the 4th was one of the busiest times of the year. For me, it meant standing in the front of the checkout lane, greeting people and packing away their purchased goods. I dreaded it. I dreaded it so much that it made me feel inadequate, alone, and depressed. Why did it make me feel that way? Were the emotions I was feeling just a young man's insecurity or foolish pride? Was I having delusions of grandeur? Or did it stem from some other area in my background or upbringing? I don't know why exactly, but from the minute I punched in at the time clock at that grocery store, my world seemed to stop at the precipice of a black hole. Bagging groceries for 10 minutes was like an hour; an hour felt like six, and a day's shift was eternity. My only lifeline during each work shift was the lawfully required breaks. I subsisted from one break to the next.

I may not have been born with immense talent, glamorous looks, supreme intelligence, or the proverbial silver spoon, but one thing I did have was friends. I had a band of really close friends that always included me in everything they did. The bond I shared with my lifelong pals was in many ways my security blanket growing up, and I am still close to all of them today. This particular 4th of July was being billed to be one for the ages for all of us. It was the first time that we all were legally old enough to be on our own. To celebrate the holiday we planned a trip to Land Between the Lakes National Recreation Area, and everyone was going. It was going to be epoch. This experience meant water skiing all day, lying out by the pool, hitting the town all night, forsaking sleep all together and living large the entire holiday weekend. Our band-of-brothers had planned this outing for some time. A few of the posse were going to go a day early and scout out the area. The rest of us would go down after I got off work the next night. So, there I was working at the end of the checkout lane, bagging customers' groceries. I had a day of work before I embarked on my weekend soiree. I detested the very idea that I was stuck in this stupid grocery store. I knew I was going to become more than this. I had to. This was no kind of life for me, stuck inside this 35,000 square foot box full of stocked shelves, weird smells, and artificial lighting, all quaintly arranged to make the establishment stakeholders rich.

I stood behind the cashier wearing the required uniform, consisting of a dress shirt, tie, and clerk apron. I grabbed cans, bread, cookies, sodas, beer, cigarettes, meats, and every single item in the store as it came off the conveyor belt. I would then hasten to sort and stuff it all into brown paper bags, load it into a grocery cart for the customers, then push it out to the parking lot and load the bags into their cars. All the while, I'd tell myself this was a job for monkeys or robots; it entailed absolutely no thought whatsoever. To make matters worse, this company paid me a menial wage. While I was doing this hapless work, my mind wondered if this was how it was going to be for me. No way! Even though I was somewhat misdirected at this time in my life, I was determined to graduate college and to somehow figure this thing out — I was unwavering in my quest to make a substantial amount of money. I just needed a chance.

As I drifted back to my present reality of packing groceries, and the drudgery of my momentary existence, something unexpected happened. Within a split-second, the mental course I had been travelling based on my choices and circumstances was about to change. Three of my friends (Billy D., Billy G., and Don H.) walked into the store Saturday morning to inform me that they were anxious to get the weekend fun underway, and they would prefer to leave in short order. There was a loyalty among us that was rare. It was important to each of them to let me know their plans so that I would not feel, or be, left out. They came to tell me that they wanted to hit the road pronto. I asked who would drive down with me tomorrow after I got off work. Uniformly, they pleaded their case that most businesses were shut down for the weekend, that each of them had fulfilled their work obligations, and that they thought it was only fitting for them to visit me at work to encourage me to join them.

So, there I was at the front of the store with three of my friends in tow and two others outside egging me on to join them. It was one of those moments in my life: do I break the implicit laws of conventional behavior, or do I conform to society's norms? Should I stay or should I go? That's what I kept asking myself over and over. I stood there looking at the faces of my best buddies contemplating the consequences. How was I going to make money? What would my parents say? Did it mean that I was a loser? As I was standing there with my green apron on, the manager approached and asked me what I was doing standing around when I had groceries to bag. This was my defining moment. I looked at him square in the eyes and paused without blinking.

"Something important has come up and I'm going to have to leave," I said.

"What do you mean you have to leave?" he asked. "What's come up that is so important?" he insisted.

"It's private and I can't get into it with you."

My friends we're snickering close by as the manager forcefully bellowed, "If you leave work now you will be fired on the spot and will never be able to work here again."

I responded confidently, "You're correct," smiled, and then walked directly past him towards the arrogant jerk in the stocking department. I walked straight up to him and tossed my apron into his arms and said, "This is for you." I turned around and walked out the door.

By closing that door, I forced my hand to play whatever fate had in store for me next. I quit, plain and simple. There was an element of reserve, even self-contempt, because my dad's friend had gotten me the job. I appreciated the gesture, but the place wasn't for me. I had far more belief in myself than working as a bagger for a national grocery store chain. Chain is exactly what that job was, a ball and chain to nowhere. I quit and never looked back. I also learned an invaluable lesson: if I find myself engaged in a job that doesn't stimulate me, it is okay to change. For me, it isn't quitting if it isn't my passion; it is simply changing. Life is short and for me to live it to the fullest, I find it essential to work in a field and environment that challenges and stimulates me at the same time. For three decades I've been working in the world of finance, which is my passion. I believe passion in our field of work is essential to living a fulfilling life. To me, settling for a paycheck was a self-sellout. No one said following our dreams would be easy, but I've found it to be worth it. The choice to join my friends on that Saturday in July ended up being one of my all-time favorite weekends. In reflection, I've found that for my internal compass to point true, I must take uncharted steps and risks at times. It is during these periods of uncertainty that I sense destiny plays a pivotal role in my life, as long as I hold on tight.

Am I proposing that quitting is okay? In specific circumstances, I am. I don't believe that everything is suited for everyone. We are all unique. My advice is to examine the situation from all sides, seek outside guidance, listen to that intuitive voice inside you, trust your instincts, and cater to your innate strengths. There are times—unexpected or critical times—when we must finish the task at hand no matter how tough the road ahead or how weathered we are from the journey. During a life-altering situation, we need to press on even if it takes us beyond our personal breaking point.

I had made a commitment to myself, more of a vow actually, to finish the Wild Sebastian 100; this time quitting wasn't an option. To quit this race after falling short at the Grand Tetons would be abject failure. Fighting my way through the agony and discomfort of running and finishing my first 100 miles was my own self-inflicted rite of passage. My family would prefer I not push the way I do. I could easily invest the time I've committed to the world of endurance sports elsewhere. Ultra-running, particularly the 100 mile distance, is what you might call an underground activity. Few people believe that running 100 miles is even possible, and many contend that it is insanity. The only opinion that mattered to me about finishing the Wild Sebastian 100 ultramarathon was my own. Could I do it? Running a 100-miler was a new and different fork in the road for me. The endurance road I had been travelling was a tough one. For some unknown reason, I kept opting to raise the bar to another level. Wild Sebastian proved to be unquestionably tougher than anything I'd previously undertaken in the endurance world. It was extremely difficult and incalculably painful, and those last 20 miles felt never-ending. I didn't quit. I finished the race. I proved to myself that I could do it.

CHAPTER 11:

Badwater 135 - The World's Toughest Foot Race

"In racing ultramarathons, you need to be humble. This sport is about improving, not winning. You never learn from winning."
—Killian Jornet (Ultramarathoner)

Badwater 135 is a 135-mile ultra-marathon (five back-to-back marathons of 26.2 miles) through Death Valley, California in the middle of July, with temperatures exceeding 120 degrees on a daily basis. Badwater 135 is considered "the world's toughest footrace." The temperature alone is enough to crush any runner's spirit, but the course itself is brutal. The race begins at the lowest point in the United States, Badwater Basin, which is 282 feet below sea level, and finishes at Mt. Whitney portal, at 8,000 feet above sea level. In essence, Badwater 135 is a perpetual, gradual incline.

Acquiring an invitation to run the race is no small feat. Each athlete needs to have an extensive history of ultra-marathon and/or endurance sports achievement, consisting of specific, verifiable, 100 mile or longer distance ultra-marathons. (For perspective, according to *Ultrarunning Magazine*, only 6,200 people have completed a running event at the 100-mile distance). Secondly, it's advised that each participant has had previous hands-on experience as a crew member at Badwater 135. And lastly, the athlete would have been wise to have participated in other Badwater branded races as a prerequisite to submitting his or her entry.

The application itself is a doozy. The requested information includes an athlete's background and history; verifiable race results and times; professional background; personal attestation of why a runner would like to run the race; and a current, or former Badwater racer that the applicant finds inspiring. The application process is akin to the college submission process with the credentials based on one's physical accomplishments, as well as one's ability to dig deep.

After completing Wild Sebastian 100 in 2013, I went on to complete a host of hundred mile races: Woodstock Festival 100 in Michigan; Keys 100, which ventured from Key Largo to Key West; Leadville Trail 100 in Colorado; Javelina Jundred 100 in Arizona; The Great New York 100 in New York City; and the Brazil 135 on the Caminho da Fe in South Brazil. They were all grueling and challenging in their regards, due to heat, elevation, and technical trails. I had also completed more 50k and 50 mile races. My running bio was getting up there and I had my sights on running Badwater. The prior year, I participated as a crew member in the Badwater 135 race, and I hoped to get my chance to run it. I knew what I was in for when I applied for entry into the race, and if I got accepted I was ready to tackle it! You could say that I was beginning to get the hang of ultramarathon racing and having a lot of fun partaking in the ultramarathon community too.

I was driving my car when the email came through on my iPhone in February, confirming that I was to be accepted into "the world's toughest footrace." I was ecstatic at the idea that I would be running Badwater, and at the same time terrified. I had been training hard for over a year with my ultramarathon coach, Lisa, in the hopes that I would be one of the 100 runners from around the world to be accepted. Now that my dream had become a reality, I had five months to get into Badwater shape, as I was determined to show up in Death Valley come July, prepared.

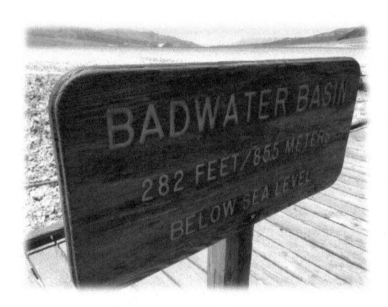

Badwater Training Schedule

To put my training in perspective, a typical training week leading up to the Badwater 135 race consisted of the following: running, tire-pulling, bridge repeats, speed-work, swimming, cycling, sauna/heat acclimation, strength and flexibility training. I would average about 4 hours per day preparing for Badwater.

A typical training week consisted of and was not limited to the following:

Weekly Training Load

➢ 60 miles of running	➢ 25 miles of cycling
➢ 20+ mile run Saturday	➢ 10 miles of tire pulling
➢ 10+ mile run Sunday	➢ 7 hours of bridge repeats
➢ 4 hours in the sauna	➢ 3 hours of hot yoga
➢ 1 hour swim	➢ 1 hour weights
➢ 1 hour calisthenics	➢ 7 hours sleep
➢ Weekly massage	➢ Biweekly acupuncture

The Journey to Death Valley

I was meticulous about having the essentials for the race. Our team would be travelling 135 miles through the desert and mountains in the middle of nowhere. Cellular service in Death Valley is sketchy at best and non-existent otherwise. There would be only three stops to fuel, add ice, beverages, and anything else. Death Valley is governed by the National Park Service. It is preserved in its natural pristine state, located in Nevada and eastern California, encompassing an area of over 3.3 million acres. Athletes and crew alike are privileged to adventure in such a place. The remote status required us to manage all the equipment needed to sustain our team of four crew members and one runner. It was our duty to clean up after ourselves. All teams were responsible for bagging and toting out all rubbish, including excrement in Biffy Bags. If crews did not have Biffy Bags, they were not allowed to participate in the race.

The list of items vital to properly race Badwater is substantial. For starters, there are clothes, shoes, tools, equipment, charts, maps and many other must-haves, adding up to over 200 items. This does not include food, ice, or hydration. Packing all of this into a van so that four crew members and one runner can function optimally is an engineering feat. It necessitates scrupulous attention to detail. Being ready for the race is an organizational phenomenon. Our team arrived two days prior to the race start, which is customary for this event. The first day is to acclimate and rest from cross-country travel. The second day is devoted to race check in and meetings, van set-up, and group photographs.

Badwater 135 has three different time wave starts: 8:00 p.m., 9:30 p.m., and 11 p.m., with the elite runners starting last. Adapting to the time differential was another wrinkle that had me uneasy. I was scheduled to start with the 8 p.m. wave, which my biological clock interpreted as 11 p.m., coming from the Eastern Time Zone. I wondered to myself how I was going to be able to stay awake for two nights in a row under Badwater's extreme environmental conditions. I reasoned that each of my fellow competitors was in the same boat as me, so I would just deal with it.

Monday, July 18, 2016 was race day. I laid low and rested while my crew prepped the van for the days ahead. My mantra was stay calm. I meditated, slept and read *Running on Empty,* by legendary ultra-runner Marshall Ulrich. The book was just what I needed to relax, and at the same time keep my head in the game. I felt well throughout the day. I ate healthy food, drank ample amounts of water, elevated my legs up the wall, and slept in the hotel room with the curtains drawn. We were set to leave for the start of the race at 7 p.m. The 17-mile drive to Badwater Basin would take us a half an hour. That would leave me 30 minutes to weigh-in, secure the GPS for the race, join the pre-race photo, and then prepare myself to run. I was very calm prior to leaving our hotel. I gathered our team for a final pre-race huddle. We said a prayer and read "If" by Rudyard Kipling—one of my father's favorite poems—and then we left.

As to be expected, the race start area was a buzz. Most of the runners were in a reserved state. The temperature was 110 degrees, with sustained 20 mph south-southwest winds that felt like a jet engine blow dryer. Oh boy, I thought, this is going to be a demanding event for all the runners and their crew. You could see the angst on everyone's faces. The first wave had approximately 30 runners all lined up for the camera. After a few snapshots, the national anthem played, and then the race began. From the onset, I took to the front. As I was exiting the staging area, I saw Coach Lisa and hastened to give her a hug. She said, "Go get 'em kid." I went on my way.

Mile 1, 2, 3... It was happening; I was officially racing the infamous Badwater 135. According to the rules, I would run the first 42 miles to Stove Pipe Wells without a pacer. My crew would be supporting me the whole time, but I'd be alone running on the road, except for other racers. We headed north for the first 17 miles. I watched the sunset over the mountain range to the west. I was mesmerized as the giant orange ball-of-fire retreated over the crest of the mountain top. It was surreal seeing the amber glow remaining for a few minutes more, before it was gone.

During races, nightfall is normally the time we put on our headlamps to illuminate our pathway. On this night in July, the full moon shone so bright that artificial lighting was unnecessary. Looking directly into the moon's ray was blinding. I ran the first

10 miles effortlessly. It normally takes me hours to settle down and fall into my running rhythm, but this night my flow came sooner. I felt good: strong, sturdy, and alert. There were a few runners jockeying back and forth with me towards the front. My game plan was to run eight minutes and then walk/recover for two minutes, and to repeat this routine as long as I held up.

The first timing station was at Furnace Creek, mile 17.6. I checked-in and kept moving. My crew was executing to perfection. There was a mutual respect amongst all of us — it was all for one and one for all. I wanted to lead my team by example in one way, but rely on them completely in another. Badwater is a team sport—the better the teamwork, the better the outcome. The hours were passing and so were the miles. Once I reached the first marathon (mile 26.2), the ebony of night with its abundance of stars and planets summoned me to pick up the pace.

As each runner advanced their mileage, their crew would provide them support, then drive a mile or two ahead and wait for the runner. This process repeated itself until the finish line. The cars pulling up next to me, some passing ahead every few miles, was distracting. I knew I needed to stay within myself and on plan, because I had roughly 100 miles still to go; nevertheless, the cars were getting into my head. I decided to pick up my running speed and pull away from the caravan of 8 p.m. runners, once and for all.

I was all business. My focus was laser-like: every stride, breath taken, and sip of fluids ingested was orchestrated. I'd run eight minutes, recover for two, meet my crew every few miles, and carefully watch my step so I did not fall. Mile 35, 40, it was happening. And then, I felt an urge. This impulse would require a lavatory. I was two miles from Stove Pipe Wells, the next time station, where there would be bathrooms. I set my mind on getting there — two miles. But my system was not having it; I was at that critical point.

Apprehensively, I flagged down my crew and told them my predicament. They said, "Go now!" I was annoyed. I couldn't believe I was going to behave like a coyote in the desert. I grabbed the things we use for such occurrences, walked into the vast desert with my Coleman lantern, turned it off, and proceeded. Hastily, I made it all happen. When I delivered the tightly sealed, double-bagged package to my crew, I took off running again, this time lighter.

Stovepipe Wells

I was relieved to arrive at Stovepipe, mile 42, with one-third of the race behind me. After running for 8 hours and 23 minutes, I had made it to the distance in the race where pacers could accompany runners. Steven Donchey, M.D., my lifelong friend, Leadman, and fellow Ironman triathlete, would be my pacer for the next several hours. I was 93 miles from the finish line, and ready to begin the first major ascent to Townes Pass. The climb begins at sea level and peaks at 4,956 feet of elevation. It was nighttime as I began the uphill climb. The heat became less of a burden as I ascended to higher elevation.

I was calm and settled knowing that Steve had my back. We had ventured together on countless endurance events, and he'd been my medical advisor always. The pacer was mandated to stay behind the runner at all times, which prevented the racer from drafting or gaining advantage. After running a few hundred feet of elevation, I backed off to power-walk the climb and conserve energy. The power-walking was rejuvenating me, and having Steve accompany me was uplifting. I wanted to log as many miles as possible before the scorching sun appeared. At an elevation of 1,000 feet, I felt considerably recovered, and with that, I began running up Townes Pass. At this juncture, the vehicles of the elite runners who started the race at 11 p.m. were starting to pass me. Car #1, Pete Kostelnick, was there first. Pete had won the race the previous year and looked to be the man to beat in 2016. As I was moving up the incline, I asked Pete's crew if he was leading and they said, "Yes." The ascent was steep with an average grade of 7.3 percent. At this point, I turned around and was moving backwards up the hill for two reasons: my coach said that it would utilize different muscles; hence, relieve the most used muscles; and primarily to watch Kostelnick make his charge. It was like having front row seats to the main event. I watched Pete and his pacer move up the climb in strides that looked effortless. I cheered him on as he made his way up towards me and even asked him how he was feeling. "I feel great!" he said. In a flash, Pete went by and vanished out of sight. I was inspired to be part of a race with some of the world's top elites.

147

I had started the race three hours before the 11 p.m. elite wave, and now the leading runners were catching up to me. Approximately 10 minutes after I reached the 1,000 foot elevation mark, another runner and his pacer passed me. I was feeling normalized and upbeat as this unknown runner moved ahead. I couldn't help noticing how efficient and precise this runner's gait appeared. I had no idea who he was, or which wave he started in, but I was amazed by the control and consistency of his stride; this guy, from my viewpoint, looked totally dialed-in. I decided to tag along for a while. This procession went on for the next hour plus. During this stretch, friends crewing for other elites were encouraging me and telling me that I was looking strong. I continued running apace with the mystery runner. At one point, my friend David Green, who was supporting an elite-wave runner, informed me that I was running with Carlos Sa, the 2013 Badwater Champion from Portugal. I couldn't believe that I was running with one of the best ultra-runners in the world, and having fun doing it. This period of the race was poetic to me. All around me as far as I could see was vast desert and mountains so grand that I felt like a speck in the universe. I felt alive; my awareness heightened to the max, but at the same time, I was mentally calculating the amount of effort I was expending running up that hill, and pondering if I should back off. At 4,000 foot elevation, there was a parking lot where the support vans were stationed. Sa and company met up with their support van and I ventured on.

I was in a zone. I had been running with Steve for over an hour and was tiring; after a few minutes I transitioned into my power walk to calm it all down. I had trained 18 months for this race and all that effort seemed to be working for me. The top runners were passing me one at a time. Being part of it all, watching each elite putting themselves on the line and pushing it to the limit, was motivating. I traded places back and forth a couple of miles with the women's champion, Ali Venti, before she left me in the dust. Never for a second did I think I would stay with any of these pros, but I sure did relish the moments alongside them, even if they had started 3 hours after I did.

After climbing uphill for the better part of 17 miles with 5,000 feet of elevation gain, I was glad to have it behind me. In no time at all, the direction became 100% downhill for the next 10 miles with an elevation loss of 3,000 feet. My coach had cautioned me to hold back on this descent so that I wouldn't blow out my quads. Craig Martin was my pacer during this descent. Craig has been a world class athlete most of his adult life, and a former Olympian for the New Zealand equestrian squad. It was fantastic having my friends there with me. The view running down towards Panamint Springs was breath-taking: a winding mirage of desert and road that seemed to go on forever. The heat was picking up for every thousand feet of elevation I descended. Running down this hill required me to be aware of every step, as falling was not something I wanted to contend with. I paid close attention to every step I took, all the way to the bottom. A couple of hours flew by, and then I was at the last five-mile section preceding Panamint Springs. The sun was baking once again. With three miles left to go before reaching the next check-in, one of my running heroes Oswaldo Lopez, a former Badwater Champion, caught up with me. Oswaldo wasn't feeling his best. I chatted with him for just a few minutes and then Dr. Donchey spoke with him.

I was looking forward to arriving at Panamint where I'd planned on eating some real food, drinking a cold beverage, icing my burning feet, and catching my breath. Thirty minutes later, I arrived at mile 72.3 with 62.7 more to go. The crew was there waiting to give me a large chocolate milkshake. The year prior, during my crewing experience I drank down two whole milkshakes; they were good. As soon as I arrived, I drank it down. The shake immediately gave me a boost. At this point in the race I had been running for 15 hours and 26 minutes, and my average pace was 12 minutes and 48 seconds per mile.

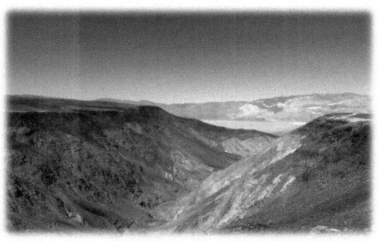

Father Crowley's Turnout

The next eight miles were back up the mountain to Father Crowley's Vista Point (mile 80). With the 120 degree heat bearing down on me and the lack of sleep adding up, I was in for a tough spell. There were several runners around me as I made my way up this winding road. Instinctively, I knew we were all giving this race our best shot. For the next five miles, I would pass and repass the same runners. I didn't care what was happening; I just needed to keep moving forward. With two miles to reach the top of this segment, I hit a wall. The heat and fatigue were tearing me down. After informing my crew of my physical state, we all agreed I should take a rest.

Ludi and Andre Chaves were the husband and wife team on my crew. They had previously crewed me at the Leadville 100 and are two of the best ultra-runners in the game. As for supporting me, they seemed to have a sixth-sense to read my mind. If I wanted, needed, or wasn't sure what was going on, they'd figure it out. I was elated to be lying down in a cool environment. I could have slept there for days, but Ludi opened the door and said, "Let's go." I asked how long I was asleep. "Ten minutes," she said. And just like that, I was out the door of the vehicle and moving back up the road. I was relieved when I eventually made it to the top of Father Crowley Lookout. The vista overlooking the valley is spectacular; we all took in the splendor. My crew could tell I was pretty beat up, so they offered assistance. Ludi set up the ice tray and in went my aching feet. She massaged my legs back to life with her healing touch, and within minutes I was back on my way.

Darwin Turn-off (mile 90.6) was the next destination, and with it was another 1,000 feet of vertical climb. After Darwin, the course would slope downward and then level out for an extended period. I was back at it. Run, walk, jog, drink, ice, and take Endurolytes and anti-fatigue tablets: repeating it all on a continuing basis. Those 10 miles were a blur. My crew kept me going in my self-induced fog state as I clicked off the miles. When I saw time station #4 in the distance, I was elated. I couldn't believe that I had just covered 10 miles. It was as if I had fallen asleep and been transported.

I had been racing for 21 hours when I asked my crew the time. They informed me that it was approximately 5:00 p.m. My next goal was to hit the 100-mile mark in under 24 hours. My fastest 100-miler was 23 hours and 23 minutes; I wanted to log a sub-24 at Badwater if possible. My crew told me that I could do it; I believed them. Then, Ludi chimed in and said, "The only way to go sub-24 is to get that ass moving." It was the funniest thing I'd heard; I took off laughing and running at the same time. Craig was running with me during this stretch, and he knew my goal of sub-24 hours. He encouraged me to pick up the pace. My mind was set and demanded my body cooperate. We were moving well and passing slower runners. A race official said that I was getting close to the 100-mile mark. The road was on a decline, and I decided to press it. I dropped my pace down to 7:30 per mile and held on until

Craig informed me that we'd made it. I passed the 100-mile mark in 23 hours and 10 minutes.

I'm sure that extra push took something out of me. I had never raced Badwater before and didn't have the experience to gauge myself precisely. The next town was Keeler (mile 108), and I was pleased when Keeler came and went. I was 14 miles away from Lone Pine (mile 122), the home of time station #5. I knew this stretch well from my prior year's crewing duties; it was the last hurdle into the town that I would be staying in after the race. Andre had been my pacer for a number of hours; his running talent and presence gave me confidence. Craig's job was to march me into Lone Pine and time station #5 at Dow Villa Motel. We made it! The routine once again was soaking my feet in an ice tray to sooth them, and quenching my thirst. As I sat down, Arthur Webb introduced himself. Mr. Webb is a decorated Badwater veteran and holds the course record for the 70 and older age group. He told me I was doing well for a rookie and to stay with it. I walked down the street and then made that final turn up Whitney Portal Road. I was 13 miles away from finishing this feat.

Whitney Portal Road

The final push would be from Lone Pine (elevation 3,700 feet) to Whitney Portal (elevation 8,371 feet). It was one o'clock in the morning; I was a shell of myself. As I trudged up the mountain, I was bottoming out. My eyes were closing; my head was spinning.

I could no longer function in a normal state. I had been at this for 29 straight hours and the sleep deficit and absolute exhaustion had taken over my resolve. I made Dr. Steve aware of my condition, and collectively the crew agreed it was best for me to take a short break. Crawling on to the van floor was painful. My legs were swollen and my feet ached and tingled. I was wired at the next level. I needed to fall asleep, but my adrenalin was too high and my mind was spinning. I was almost at the end, but I wasn't. I fell asleep. Ten minutes later, the door opened, and I stumbled out of the van and back on to the course. Three miles after my last break, I had to do it again: lie down, close my eyes, and sleep for another 10 minutes.

I had given this race my all, and I wanted it over. My crew supported me nonstop, and I felt bad keeping them out there with seven miles to go. Two miles later, I was busted again. My vision became so blurry that I could not see. My eyes were watering profusely. Walking was rickety, and I felt as if I was about to collapse. I went back in the 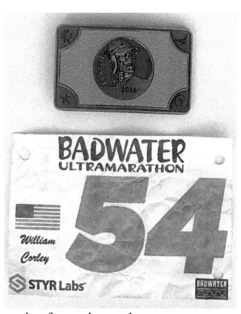 van and this time I was able to arise four minutes later on my own. The third time was a charm: I felt awake. Steve and I listened to

Jackson Brown on my external speaker, reminiscent of our college days. The music perked me up. I passed the last check-in at 4 a.m. with three miles of the climb remaining.

In customary fashion, my crew and I crossed the finish line together; we were greeted by Chris Kostman, the Badwater Race Director. It was over. We arrived at the finish line, mile 135, at 5:25 a.m., 33 hours and 25 minutes after the journey began.

Friendship

*"I would rather walk with
a friend in the dark, than alone in the light."*
—Helen Keller

What fueled my career and athletic pursuits? Friendship! Whenever I undertake an endurance race that pushes me past my limits, I try to ascertain what I learned from the experience. I was pleased with my performance at Badwater. I'd trained for a decade in the endurance world; my output at Badwater was a byproduct of all those years of hard work, discipline, and focus. The race taught me that I wasn't alone in my endeavors.

A few years prior to Badwater, I raced my second 100-mile race in Pinckney, Michigan amidst rainy and nasty weather; there was even a tornado. Around mile 90, a pack of five ultra-runners grouped together. This wasn't by design: it was by chance, and we instinctively began working as a unit. By working, I mean that we were giving one another moral support. The tie that bonded us at this point in the race was pain. We had 10 miles to go to finish the race, and after running for over 24 hours, our feet and bodies hurt badly. It was at this point that I wondered why I was doing this to myself. No one was making me go through this pain fest; I didn't get paid for it, and I had already proven to myself that I could do it. Then and there, at mile 90, I asked the other runners in the pack why they were running 100 miles. I wasn't going to tell them my answer until I heard theirs. One by one, I conducted my survey. What astonished me was that every one of us had the same exact answer. We weren't there trying to find our true selves, or to see how much we could endure; nor were we trying to find enlightenment or anything of the sort. The answer was — we did not know. We were running for over 24 hours, and not one of us had any idea why. We all laughed out loud at this coincidence, while still grimacing in pain. Certainly, something was drawing us to it, but we didn't know what.

There have been times in my life when I lost my way and felt isolated. I read a quote once that went something like this, "You have to be a little lost, before you can find what you're looking for." The words resonated with me. At times I can be too hard on myself and become my worst enemy.

As a teenager, I wanted to be part of the in-crowd. I wasn't a banner student. My athletic talent was marginal. Physically, I was a late bloomer. I always looked young for my age. I compensated for my flimsy self-esteem through humor. I noticed that if I could make others laugh, it opened doors for me. I was a good-natured kid. I was known to be competitive if interested in a specific activity, subject, or person. I liked to win. Lucky for me, a top college quarterback moved from another state to my town and agreed to train me as a future quarterback. According to him, I had a pretty strong throwing arm and reasonable instincts. So, I practiced the drills to play quarterback for months on end, and by the time high school tryouts started, I was ready to give it a shot. I actually believed I could make the squad as a backup quarterback. I wasn't gunning for the top spot—my friend Blair had the starting

QB position wrapped up, and he was a top-notch collegiate prospect. I never let him know that I was trying out for QB, because I didn't want him to mock me. I didn't even care if I got second string; I just wanted to play QB. The first day of tryouts, the coach lined all the high school players up and barked out the command, "Lineman go here, linebackers go there, running backs with the running back coach, quarterbacks with the QB coach, defensive backs go over there, and kickers stay put."

I watched all of the athletes go towards their respective positions, while I hesitated. There were many athletes going to each of the positions, but only two went for QB. I looked at them. They were naturally-gifted athletes; I couldn't even imagine myself competing against them. I wilted within myself and walked over to the defensive backs. I was scared to death of what the other athletes would say if I joined the two QBs, so I went to the defensive back group. I dumped my dream of being a quarterback then and there, for all the wrong reasons. I was disappointed in myself. I learned a valuable lesson that day, but it took years for me to understand it.

What's the lesson in all this, and how is it related to financial well-being? In order to get my act together along my life's journey, I had to learn from my past mistakes. The lesson that I learned during my football tryouts helped me with my decision to become an entrepreneur. The competitive side of me believed that I could do better financially by making my own decisions. Working for a large company, it wasn't hard to figure out that managers had their favorites and cronies. All businesses have people in charge who have their own way of doing things and their unique personalities and norms. I was okay with most of that, even if my manager was an unjust, self-adulating, backwards-thinking blockhead. My job was to generate revenue for the company and myself. I didn't get involved with inner office politics and gossip. I was focused on making money; yet, the system had reach and tentacles that affected me professionally and personally. If I was working harder than someone else and outperforming them in all metrics, but they were somehow getting perks to grow their business that I deserved, it didn't sit well with me. If I earned it, I wanted it. I performed well enough in the corporate world that I had developed the confidence necessary to believe that I could succeed on my own, and that's what I did. I left and opened my own brokerage firm.

I had built a reputation as a producer and the word was getting around that other financial advisors would join me right away, but that rumor proved false. In the end, it was just me. Previously, I invested in an accounting firm, and I was able to use its offices to launch my investment firm. Having other associates around me was good in some ways, but in reality, I was completely on my own. I remember the pressure I was under to provide for my family. Sending three kids to private school is costly. While setting up the company, I wasn't earning any money. I had to make money in short order. I worked around the clock; I produced, managed, administered, planned, dealt with problems, and provided compliance for the firm.

The first year the pressure was so intense that it was not uncommon for me to lie down on the floor next to my desk around noon and pass out. I never planned these naps, but I literally couldn't hold my head up. Back then, I was also a junk-food aficionado, which didn't help matters. I remember panicking and questioning my decision to leave a high paying job as a Vice President at Merrill Lynch, one of the nation's premier brokerage houses. Now, I was trying to figure out how to make ends meet. It was a low point that I kept inside.

In a year's time, the company I founded started to gain traction. Sales and profits increased, and with it came more tasks and responsibilities. I was accustomed to depending only on myself. People who knew me said that I could be controlling at times. That's not how I wanted to be, yet ultimately the failure or success of the company fell on my shoulders. I trained employees, but they were young and inexperienced. I needed some additional seasoned professionals to take on some of the load. It took a few years before things finally came together, and I found the right people. Not only did I get the right managers to join me, many of them remain with me to this day. Each of my colleagues is a conscientious, intelligent, hardworking team player, and trusted friend. I've grown to rely on them 100% and believe they do the same with me.

In college, I took a Psychology class where I learned about Abraham Maslow's Hierarchy of Needs. I am blessed to say that my basic needs were always provided for by my family. My psychological needs entailing belonging, love, and self-esteem occasionally fell short. At the top of Maslow's pyramid is self-actualization. Self-actualization is about reaching one's full potential creatively, personally, and professionally. I see self-actualization more like a process than a goal. I believe that we can all grow, evolve, and become better or higher versions of ourselves. Not only do I think we can, I believe we must. I know in my case it is the only way. Self-actualization is that voice inside me that strives for me to become more than I am. I am my own judge and jury. Striving for self-actualization and its attainment are the building blocks and foundation of my self-esteem.

Throughout our lives, the better we become and the more successful we are, the greater our responsibility is to make a positive impact in the world. Life and its rewards come with obligations. Personally, I have a faith that guides me from within. My faith is based on loving principles. It is about me doing for others as I would like others to do for me. However, I still have bouts of self-doubt, short-comings, and inner tribulation. I believe that working through dark days is a part of life. I have tools that I use whenever I am feeling down. Talking is one of my favorite tools; talking to a friend lessens the load. I've found that my true friends have many of the same reservations, and conversing with one another helps each of us find our way back. My inspiration often comes from people. There are moments and days when I feel all alone. Even if I am hitting it on all cylinders, I sometimes lose my way.

I can remember special events when everyone was festive and gleeful; I was with loved ones and friends and everything was fine, but I felt disconnected and isolated. Reality isn't always a bed of roses for me, and I doubt it is for anyone. America is a great country, but it takes a tremendous amount of effort for most of us to live out the American dream. I've seen ups and downs, high points and low points. I've experienced them physically, mentally, emotionally, and spiritually. To me, it's all part of being human.

The lesson that was reinforced during my Badwater experience was further confirmation that I am not alone. I don't have to have it all figured out. I am learning to let go more often and to trust in others more wholeheartedly. During the race, I had to rely on my supporting cast. They took total responsibility for me running the race to completion. In my work, I have others that I depend on. My family and friends are my most important support. I need to connect with each of these people to be part of the whole. At the same time, I have to learn to be alone and to keep growing as a man and member of the human race. I feel centered more often than not these days, but I'm sure I will lose my way again. It's okay though, because I know that I have others to lean on, and hobbies, outlets, discoveries, and new beginnings ahead of me. It's taken me most of my life, but I'm learning not to take myself so seriously. I can laugh at myself. Even though it doesn't always feel like it, I am not alone. I believe humans need to love and to be loved. Of all the things I've written about in this book, I would say friendship is most important.

CHAPTER 12:

After Badwater - Summiting Mount Whitney

*"The only way to discover the limits of the possible
is to go beyond them to the impossible."*
—Arthur Clarke (Writer)

The peak of Mount Whitney stands as the highest point in the continental United States. It is located in Inyo National Forest, in Eastern Sierra Nevada, California. It is a majestic place full of birds, marmots, giant sequoias/redwoods, flowing streams, alpine lakes, spires, granite cliffs, and its crest is capped with snow and ice. Most hikers that ascend this one-of-a-kind mountain commence their journey from Whitney Portal, which sits at an elevation of approximately 8,000 feet. It is an eleven-mile trek from Whitney Portal to the mountain's peek, with over 6,000 feet of elevation gain. Attempting this ascent and descent turnaround of 22 miles is considered an extreme day hike. To grasp the difficulty of this hike, a typical person walking through their shopping mall will average around a 20 minute per mile pace (3 miles per hour). Individuals planning a one day turn around on Mount Whitney will likely begin the journey before sunrise, and finish the trip some 12 to 18 hours later, depending on their experience, physical status, and weather conditions, which is an average pace somewhere between 30 to 50 minutes per mile. After finishing Badwater, it was customary for the pioneers of the race to complete the final leg of the journey to the summit of Mt. Whitney the following day.

The final push covers the Mount Whitney Trail, from the trailhead at 8,350', to the mountain summit at 14,505', and back to trailhead, a roundtrip of 22 miles. My ultimate goal was to finish off those 22 miles, if I was physically capable after racing Badwater.

Mount Whitney 14,505 Feet

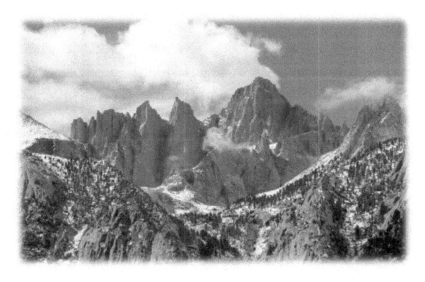

I set the alarm to go off at 4:30 a.m. After sleeping for less than five hours the past three days, I questioned my ability to attempt this feat. My body was trashed from the 135 miles I'd just put myself through. When the alarm rang, I sat up and gingerly shifted my legs off the bed and onto the floor. I made my way to the wash basin and brushed my teeth; I was a moving zombie. My friend Dr. Donchey was there with me, and he too was significantly sleep deprived. We were completely silent; we were saving all of our energy so that we could make climbing up Mt.

Whitney a reality. After organizing ourselves mentally, we met my pal Craig in the lobby and the three of us headed out the door. We quickly picked up some food and drinks to consume along the way and drove the 13 miles to the Whitney Portal Trailhead. It was still dark out just before 6 a.m. when we hit the trail. My mind was awash with uncertainty. I wanted to make this summit part of my story; it meant that I could be a part of Badwater folklore. When I set out on this mission, the first thing I had to do was finish the 135-mile race in the desert. Now that I had Badwater behind me, I had one more hurdle to go: reaching Whitney Summit.

The first couple miles of hitting the trail, I felt physically deficient. I was the weakest link and did not want to have my friends waiting for me. I directed my friends to carry on at their own pace and to no longer wait for me. We had walkie-talkies that transmitted for miles, so I knew that we would be able to communicate for the most part (although, there were places along the route where the mountains blocked the signal). I'd summited the mountain twice the year before. I'd gone up initially solo, and again two days later with fellow ultra-runner and Renaissance man Bradford Lombardi, but never in my current state. As I watched my pals march off in front of me, I felt somewhat uneasy and alone initially, but I regained my composure as I moved up the mountain. Movement, I've found, invariably changes my state. No matter what my mood is or what's on my mind, there's always a positive shift in my energy after I get up and move. In many instances, I've observed the more deliberate the movement, the more pronounced the shift. Whenever I find myself in a sullen state, motion has become my go-to anecdote.

For the most part, I knew my way up the trail, which gave me confidence. My body was beat-up. To complete this final hurdle, I needed to be as aware of everything going on in and around me as possible. Looking, walking, stepping, eating and drinking were my only points of concentration. I tried to keep it all as simple as possible. The scenery on the mountain was majestic, but I was only taking it in at a cursory level. My focus was on staying alert and running my own internal diagnostics: keep moving forward, replenish and maintain my water supply from the mountain's streams and lakes, take in nourishment, rest whenever I felt light-headed or tired; and above the tree line, apply sunscreen for protection. I repeated this process continuously. I felt mentally connected by repeating each task that kept my spirits up. Every half hour, the others would contact me on their walkie-talkies to check on me; it kept me engaged.

The first few hours alone I questioned my resolve. Early that morning my body had been stiff and sore, but as the hours passed, my body responded favorably. What drove me to make this trek was the fact that others had completed this pilgrimage. That was enough to keep me driving onward. I was on my way up this beast of a mountain; I was tired, but determined. I had a long way to go, but I had my formula to succeed, which I learned from ultra-running greats: just keep moving forward. My hiking gait was wobbly and haggard. Generally speaking, I was a sight for sore eyes. I was marching up that trail like a drunkard, but at least I was going in the right direction. The miles were passing, and before long I had arrived at Trail Camp, located at mile six.

For overnighters, Trail Camp is the last designated camping area on the way up; it sits above the tree line at 12,000 feet. For day hikers like me, Trail Camp is the last respite before the pathway becomes a granite rock fest. Trail Crest was next. It was located at mile nine, it stands at 13,650 feet. Trail Crest encompasses the remaining two miles to the mountain's peak. As a rule of thumb, there is about one percent less oxygen available for every 100 meters of ascent. Pushing through those last two miles on 40% less oxygen was going to be a test. It was proving to be a slog for me; I found myself oxygen deficient every quarter mile, my head swimming from light-headedness, and I had run out of food. I knew that I'd see my friends on their switchback, but I did not know when. I was feeling the culmination of my body's fatigue with less than a mile to the top. As I reached the final ridge, I met my friends on their way back down. I was really glad to see them. They shared their provisions with me, and accompanied me to the summit. Meeting back up with them instantly lifted my spirits. I took photos, signed and dated the summit log book, and hung out for a few minutes with my pals and new friends we made at Badwater. We were standing there together at one of the highest points on the planet. The sky was crystal blue, the air clean, crisp, cool, and refreshing. Weather on the summit is fickle, but on this

July early afternoon the weather was ideal. And then, just like that, we headed back down the mountain in case the weather changed abruptly.

Nuno Castro, my friend from Portugal, and I commenced the Whitney Mountain descent together. We met a few days earlier during the Badwater race. He was a physical force, one of those rare men who are naturally strong. He had an inviting personality and soon became my protector on the way down the mountain. As I descended the rugged granite mountainside, he looked out for me the entire way. My exhaustion was now mired in unfamiliar territory. I wanted this adventure to be over—one by one I was slowly clicking off the miles. Going down the mountain is much easier than going up it, but the downward portion seems longer for some strange reason. Logically, the energy a person expends to reach the summit is a limited resource, and even though the descent is not as difficult, the fatigue factor associated with the trip to the top makes it feel longer than it actually is. Twisting, scaling, lunging, walking, jumping and slipping were all part of the descent. The mountain seemed different at every turn and familiar at the same time.

I kept anticipating the lower switchbacks near the trailhead, because my memory was telling me that that section of the trail was groomed and easier to navigate. I couldn't seem to get there. Descending the mountain was just more of the same — moving, watching each of my steps to keep from falling, and carefully planting my aching feet. I had to take extra care to protect my feet, as they were sore and tender beyond belief. Even the slightest stub against a rock or root would send me yelping. We clocked the final two miles in 45 minutes; it felt like hours. As we exited the trail and headed towards our minivan in the parking lot, I was numb. It was over. Somehow I made it. I completed the journey from Badwater Basin, the lowest point in the United States at 282 feet below sea level, to the Whitney Summit at 14,505 feet, totaling 157 miles. Now it was time to sleep!

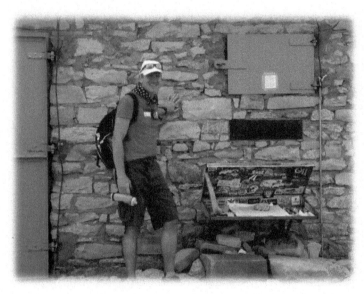

Financial Fitness

"Everyone's a genius. But if you judge a fish by its ability to climb a tree, it will live its whole life believing that it is stupid."
—Albert Einstein

Earlier in this book, I expressed my view regarding the merits of human struggle. My aim in this section is to illustrate how I have benefitted personally and grown from such occurrences. For starters, I was never one to sit idly. My mother would be the first to say that I was never the bashful type. As a teenager, you might say that I was impetuous at times. I always strived to be part of the in-crowd. Fitting in was important to me. At times, peer pressure would find me taking daring chances to gain favor with others. If I had to do it over, it's likely that the adult me would think twice about several of my adolescent decisions. Growing up, I was prone to jumping into the proverbial deep end before testing the water. In hindsight, I came to recognize my hasty actions as an outreach for approval, because deep inside me (an area I didn't know) I was insecure.

I don't always agree with society at large. I am a stand-up guy and take responsibility for my actions. But then again, I am unsure whether the rules society outlines for us to follow—the norms, the acceptances, the fitting in—make sense. I question the fabric of society and ponder whether its purpose is altruistically bent, or if it is something less noble. Living in a small town for the first eighteen years of my life, I experienced the differences between the haves and have-nots, those that had money and those that didn't. My parents worked hard to provide the best for my siblings and me, but we were far from the movers and shakers in our community; I didn't like it. It made me feel inadequate.

I was never the best at any activity of distinction, but I tried to be just the same. I conveyed a certain level of self-assuredness when it came to attempting challenging pursuits that others mostly shied away from, and I had a lively sense of humor to pep things up when necessary. At times, my bravado would get the best of me, and I'd find myself in the wrong place with the wrong people at the wrong time. During some of these instances the outcome wasn't good. Conversely, there were other times that I benefitted by stepping out, speaking up, and crossing over the line, during which my actions would achieve their objectives and even open doors.

Both my parents were well educated with graduate degrees; they set an example for me and my siblings as lifelong learners. In the early part of my life, my problem with education was that I wasn't interested in sitting through school all day and then taking the time to hit the books at night. I wanted to do things my way and on my terms, which translated into hanging out with my friends and goofing off. It wasn't until I graduated from college and had to earn a living to support myself that I had my wake-up call.

My parents worked long and hard to provide me with the best of everything they could afford on middle-class pay. The day I graduated college, my father handed me a Shell gasoline credit card and said, "Son, I am completely out of money. I've done all I can for you at this point, but I can no longer afford to support you. Use this credit card if you need it to survive. I love you." Sadly, I'd been so caught up in my own world, my selfish pleasures, my aloof attitude, that I had ignored the financial burden I'd been on my father for too long. That was it; from that point forward, I was going to get my act together and make a positive, meaningful impact in my parents' lives personally and financially. I had always loved my parents dearly, but now it was time for me to put-up or shut-up. Failing wasn't an option.

Einstein said, "All knowledge comes from experience." I had none whatsoever. My quest to become financially fit began at ground zero. I had no experience pertaining to anything in the business world, or how to make money for that matter. My knowledge was limited to my college business degree. All I had going for me was a burning desire. Desire would prove to be enough to get me started.

I view summiting Mt. Whitney as a metaphor of sorts. Each of us has mountains to climb. From the start, we begin climbing the mountain of primary and secondary education. Then there's college or specialty trade school. Next comes getting a good job and earning enough money to take care of ourselves, and later, being able to provide for our families. I think the mountain peaks keep rising higher and higher for those with enterprising spirits. By striving for even bigger and better achievements and climbing to the summit, life seems to become more meaningful.

Early in my career, I tried to make calculated decisions to put myself in winning situations. Some of these decisions proved to be more challenging than expected. I needed to make money to survive and failure wasn't an option; failure meant giving up. Instinctively, I knew that if I kept my burning desire stoked, somehow, I would make it. That burning desire meant working one extra day, one extra hour, making one extra call. Looking back on those early days when things were on the brink financially, somehow it always worked out, as if an act of providence was there when I needed it most.

Life is full of firsts. As I was building my business, my modus operandi was to always lead by example. Whether that meant working seven days a week, taking out the office rubbish, or not getting paid for weeks on end, I became accustomed to going the extra mile. One of the most difficult aspects of building a company on a shoestring budget is the acquisition and retention of key personnel. I retained my team members by treating them with admiration and respect. But even then, I had a hard time trusting others.

From the onset of filing initial documents to incorporate the company, to signing the operating lease and opening the doors for business, I always had my finger on the pulse of everything. I was the captain of the ship. I welcomed others' opinions along the way, but I needed to make all major decisions for the company. As the company grew in size, I could no longer oversee every detail. When it came down to operating and managing the business, I found it really hard to let go and trust others. It took me twenty years to clearly understand the merits of delegation.

By treating my associates as partners and going above and beyond, they stayed with me and became trusted advisors. Their commitment to the company instilled my faith and trust in them. Collectively, we have laid a foundation to build upon, a starting point from which to climb the mountain together. One thing I have learned for sure: the best way to aim and reach for the stars is with a firm foundation, and a burning desire for success to fuel the journey. And it is never too late to start from scratch!

CHAPTER 13:

Winning a 100 Miler

"80 percent of success in life comes from just showing up."
—Woody Allen

I'm not going to question the merits of Woody's cliché, but I've seen up close and personal how "just showing up" can make a difference in life. In the midst of writing this book, three months after competing in Badwater, I attempted another long distance ultra, aptly named, The Pumpkin Holler Hunnerd. Guess what? I won! How'd it happen? The best answer I can provide is that I showed up. This 100-miler was located outside of Tahlequah, Oklahoma in a 17,000 acre wildlife preserve situated in the Ozarks. As a boy, I had traveled to Tulsa by car and remembered it being completely flat. Oh boy was I wrong!

As a seasoned endurance athlete, you would think that at this stage of the game I would adequately plan and be prepared for every 100-mile ultramarathon. That would mean taking the time to familiarize myself with the course, its slope, the topography and where the place is actually located on the map. I didn't do any of it. I had no idea where I was going, how difficult the course would be, or how long it would take me to reach the starting line from the Tulsa Airport. My only planning for this race was in the training: at least I was physically prepared.

At this time, my business had been picking up steam, which is always a good thing. But, the increase in activity required me to put in more and longer work hours to effectively manage it all. Because of these demands, I chose the latest flight after work Thursday evening. As Murphy's Law would have it, the flights were delayed, and by the time I finally made it to the hotel it was past one o'clock in the morning. After sleeping in that morning, eating, shopping for racing supplies (food and drinks), driving to Tahlequah, signing in for the race at packet-pickup, organizing my drop bags, and attending the pre-race meeting, it was eight o'clock at night. The race was set to start two hours later, and I was feeling completely exhausted. I was nervous and confused about my decision to begin racing that late at night. I am just a regular person; I am no different than anyone reading this book. When I'm hungry, I eat. When I am sick, I go to the doctor. When I'm afraid, I lock the door. Additionally, when I've had a non-stop day full of activity and I've depleted my energy for the day, I go to sleep to replenish myself.

I needed sleep, and I needed it badly. My head was spinning with trepidation. In less than two hours, I was going to put a headlamp on my forehead, venture out into the middle of nowhere, and run 100 miles. The ultra-community is small, and once you've been around it awhile, it's like you know everybody. Ultra-runners attending these events travel from all over the world. I've made some good friends doing ultras, and I feel comfortable opening up to a few of them. As I was greeting my pals, I let them know the state I was in. I needed some support or realization that I was about to commence this undertaking when I was beyond exhausted. I asked my fellow ultra-runners for advice; their answers were unexpectedly fitting. They told me that they were as tired as I was. I was feeling miserable and found company that felt the same way. I actually laughed at the very idea of it all. At that moment, I realized the game was indeed on for me. I mentally crossed through the emotional block keeping me from committing to what I was about to get into. I looked at my watch and I still had enough time for an hour's nap. I immediately went back to my rental car, reclined the seat, set the alarm on my iPhone, and went to sleep.

I slept for an hour. When my alarm sounded, I had 10 minutes to get to the starting line. It was not going to happen; I was in no mood to rush. I needed to change into my running clothes, lube my feet, tape sensitive areas on my body prone to chaffing, put on my flashers and headlight, and fill my water bottle. By the time I finished all of this, the race was underway. I could not have cared less. As I moved towards the starting line my running pal Carl Hineline from Texas reminded me to pass over the timing strip to validate that I had started the race properly, which I did. I took my sweet time and wasn't putting pressure on myself. I knew that I had 100 miles to go and plenty of time to make up for my tardiness. Once I began running, I was approximately 10 minutes behind the leaders. It was pitch black as I headed out from the starting line. My steps were guided by the artificial light on my head, and the red flashers around my waist were blinking away;

my mind was blank and numb as I directed my legs and body to move.

After running at a brisk pace for just over an hour, I caught up with Carl. We both knew the demands on our bodies that come from running 100 miles. We buddied up and were running at a manageable pace. We had a long, long way to go and were under no pressure to overexert ourselves in the early going. Steady-as-she-goes was my mantra. The key for me was to keep moving forward, log the miles, and not look back. The hours were clicking by: midnight, 1:00 a.m., 2:00 a.m., 3:00 a.m., and by 4:00 a.m., I was a zombie. I was running all the flats and most of the downhills; to conserve energy, I walked the uphills. During the uphills, I was literally falling asleep as I ascended. Carl grabbed my arm several times to keep me from falling asleep on my feet. My sleep deprivation owned me. I was in a dark place, literally and figuratively.

The sleepwalking was the worst on the way up the hills. Even though my heart rate was elevated during each incline, it wasn't beating fast enough to keep me awake. I needed sunlight! The rising sun is like magic to me. No matter how sleepy I am, once the sun rises, I wake up. Sunrise in this densely wooded area would be just before 7:00 a.m. I didn't think I could make it. As I faded off during each ascent, I seriously contemplated lying down in the middle of the country road and sleeping for 20 minutes or so. But then, I'd reach the top of the hill and start running again. Running faster made my heart rate increase, and somehow, this woke me up. It was a vicious cycle. I was doing my best to hold on and stay focused in hopes that the sun would rise. Just like that, I'd find myself sleepwalking up another ascent, and then I'd reach the top and run to wake up. The remaining hours passed; finally the sun rose, and with it, my spirits.

The race comprised three 30 mile loops on mostly dirt and gravel country road, with a 16 mile out and back extension added to the initial lap. Each loop began and ended at the start-finish area, where most of the guests and support crew resided. I was running this race self-crewed. I would rely on each aid station across the course and its volunteers for my food, drink and necessities. I had been running for eight hours and my body felt achy and stiff. I finished the first 35 miles and reentered the staging area. Volunteers supporting other runners came to my aid and helped tend to my discomfort and personal requests. I desperately needed to regroup, physically and mentally. After resting and replenishing myself with caffeine, protein drinks, foot care, and crowd encouragement, I headed back out on the course. I was happy that it was daytime. It gets annoying running with a headlamp for extended hours in the dark. My vision is not what it used to be and it can be hard for me to see at night. I was determined to capitalize on the next 12 daylight hours and get as many miles under my belt as I could before nightfall ensued. By the time I hit the halfway mark, I began to feel better. My stiffness had lessened to a degree, and I was running more efficiently. I remained constant in my effort and attentive to every step. The miles were passing, and before I knew it, I was arriving at the end of the second loop with over 70 miles under my belt and 30 miles to go. Immediately, friends came to my aid. The temperature was in the high 80s and my feet were burning. Once again, I needed to regroup. This time I put my aching, burning feet into a large Ziploc bag full of ice. The icing of my feet was both uncomfortable and soothing. I had passed a lot of runners at this point and sensed I was nearing the leaders. My goal was to earn the coveted sub-24-hour belt buckle for 100 miles. I was right on target, but needed to remain vigilant. After treating my feet with ointment and putting on fresh socks, I hit the road for the last loop.

The moment I started the final loop, I analyzed and reassessed my goals. At this point in the race I was essentially racing two clocks: the first being the sun, as I wanted to get as many miles behind me before sunset; the second being the elapsed time, as I was determined to earn a 24 hour buckle. For this to become a reality, I needed to push for 30 more miles. I had no idea what place I was in at this point. I had encountered runners on the switchbacks and assumed there were three or four in front of me. I was only racing toward my own goal. I ran every descent and flat with purpose; I was pushing myself well beyond my comfort zone. The volunteers at each aid station were amazing. They gave me food, drink, ice, and electrolytes. I even drank a couple of beers with ice in my water bottle during the race. Beer has calories, carbonation, and alcohol, and for me, the combination worked. I added ice to offset the diuretic effects.

With 25 miles to go, my body was resisting the onslaught of my mental push. My knees hurt, my back was tight, my feet were swollen, and my mind was exhausted. Volunteers told me that I was running well and encouraged me. They let me know that I was near the top of the leaderboard. Although I was not concerned with my race position, it was motivating to have spectators cheer me on. At mile 80, something unusual happened. I had been running at a sub 10 minute pace for a number of miles. I kept telling myself that I'd stop and regroup at some point, and yet I wasn't stopping. And then it happened: my body passed through to another dimension. The pain seemed to have disappeared. I continued running unabated.

With 15 miles to go, the sun began to set. I had less than three hours remaining if I could hold it all together. I was mostly concerned about the throng of aggressive dogs that I'd have to pass at night. I made up my mind that I was going to run as fast as I could past them. I waited until the last minute to turn on my headlamp. I was running from the heart. At every aid station, volunteers and runners alike rooted for me to keep pressing on. I was totally focused, and yet the extreme fatigue was affecting my vision. Everything was blurry, as if I had been in a chlorinated pool swimming all day without a mask. It was then that my headlamp illuminated a poisonous water moccasin. I stumbled and screamed. I had just missed it. If I would have landed on it, it would have lit me up and how! My pulse went through the roof. It took a moment before I pulled it together and kept running.

The dogs were to be my final obstacle. As I approached the miles where the mangy canines lived, I was in the zone. At this point, I'd resigned myself to whatever was going to happen. I was not taking my focus off finishing, and getting there in short order was my

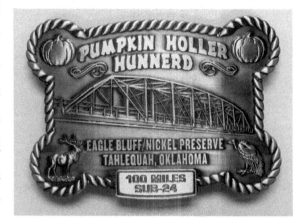

mission. As luck would have it, the dogs were a nonevent this time around. At the next-to-last aid station, I filled up my bottle with Coca-Cola and kept moving. With a mile to go, the final aid station crew cheered me on. Ten minutes later, I crossed the finish in 23 hours and 45 minutes, beating my 24 hour goal by 15 minutes. I showered outdoors, ate some great grilled food, and went to sleep for the first time in two days. When I awoke the next morning, I received a text message from Carl that I had come in first overall. I attribute my first 100 mile win at this race to just showing up and finishing.

K.I.S.S.

"The root of all evil isn't money;
rather, it's not having enough money"
—Gene Simmons (Rock Musician)

KISS is my acronym for "KEEP IT SIMPLE, <u>SAVE</u>!" The KISS principle is perhaps most vital when it comes to getting it right in business, personal finances, and even fitness. Which do you think is more important: the amount you save each year; or the amount earned on your savings and investments? If you answered the amount you save, you're correct. Saving money is crucial. Wages and salaries are subject to ever-changing market forces and individual productivity. Likewise, the returns we receive on our investments vary and are unpredictable. The amount we save each month is a personal choice that we control. The key is living below our means. Focused savings is the baseline for everyday Americans to build wealth. Keep it simple, *save*!

According to the Federal Reserve's *Report on the Economic Well-Being of U.S. Households in 2016*, 44 percent of survey respondents indicated that they do not have sufficient funds available to pay for a $400 emergency. The lack of money for nearly half of all Americans can be compared to a runaway locomotive; the only way to stop it from becoming a colossal disaster is by putting money aside, now!

Saving money is a non-starter for some folks and a lost art for countless others. There are numerous reasons why a person or business does not or cannot save money. The typical person finds saving money so difficult because expenses add up quickly: modest wage earnings, unemployment or job loss, increased shelter cost, health insurance, life insurance, automobile expenses, food, medicine, clothing, utilities, entertainment, car insurance, disability insurance, and taxes crimp everyone's discretionary income. By the time most folks tackle ongoing expenses, there isn't a whole lot left over, if any.

The same holds true for businesses (especially start-ups); they are laden with never-ending expenditures. The cost to operate a company is substantial. It costs a lot to run a business and even more to expand it. Business growth consumes cash, and fast growth consumes cash fast. Saving money requires businesses and individuals alike to be vigilant. The act of saving money is strategic.

So, what's a hardworking person to do to rectify this impasse? I've yet to find an easy remedy. But there is light at the end of the tunnel, and it is not a locomotive heading your way. It is a white light illuminating a better way to make savings happen. Whether you are just starting out or are well into your golden years, somehow you've made it this far. That's the good news. My point is that no matter what's occurred in your life, you've somehow found the means necessary to eat, sleep, live. If, however, you've found it necessary to take out loans, borrow on credit cards, and/or lease your vehicle versus purchase it, maybe it's time to take a step back and evaluate it all. Did you really need everything you've purchased up to this point?

I've found as a planner and organizer, the best way to get a handle on spending is by breaking things down into smaller pieces. In the past 24 hours, could you have saved on a purchase or expenditure? I see countless areas where people are overspending. It's obvious to most that they may be prone to small impulse items, such as Starbucks or Dunkin Donuts. It is less obvious and greater expenditures are overlooked in ongoing expenses: automobile insurance; cellular, cable, and satellite services; public utilities; taxes; and even streaming subscriptions. It is important to take the time at least once a year to scrutinize our ongoing expenditures and see if we can eliminate or lower the costs. Just yesterday, I cut loose a subscription that I no longer deemed essential (it probably never was) and will save $6.95 a month. Now, I'll invest the $6.95 into my savings and watch it grow.

Remember, it is not about how much you make, it is about how much you keep! I'm sure you've heard stories of regular folks winning the lottery or hitting it big at the casino, only to end up flat broke. No one is exempt from the perils of profligate spending. Many of the rich and famous who have earned millions but failed to govern their urges have found themselves falling on hard times. Actors, stars, and athletes such as Wesley Snipes, Kim Basinger, Curt Schilling, Larry King, M.C. Hammer, Burt Reynolds, Ulysses Grant, Mickey Rooney, and Mike Tyson made boatloads of money and all went broke. Even Lady Gaga had a bad spell sending her into bankruptcy in 2009. Each of these stars was driven more by their wants than by their needs. Ironically, most windfall recipients choose to go it alone, and fail to employ the services of reputable professional advisors to assist them with their newfound wealth. This may ultimately lead to financial ruin. Mentorship matters!

Do you know what self-defeating financial trait this cast of famous people shared? Not saving! All of them and countless others spent more money than they earned. That's right, they did not <u>SAVE.</u> Why wouldn't they save? Simply because they didn't know how or why. Saving money is not self-punishment; it is self-emancipation. Saving money is freedom from the tyranny of consumerism. Saving money is not about the accumulation of things. It is not about a life of endless leisure. Saving money is a virtue. Instead of keeping up with the Joneses, saving money portrays self-confidence. Saving money is an inner expression of "To thine own self be true." It is liberation!

Everyone wants to be financially fit and free from financial hardship. It is essential for investors to be true to themselves. I advise that you live within or below your means and save money always. Every dollar saved is a step forward. Start saving now: daily, weekly, monthly, yearly. I use the S.T.A.R. formula. Mastering this principle will not only make life more abundant, it can lead to real wealth.

S.T.A.R. investors prepare for various outcomes: inflationary and noninflationary growth scenarios. The acronym is the following: **(S)**eventy-five percent is the most, and twenty-five percent is the least, that a star investor will invest into the market at a given time. The idea is to load up on equities when values are low, and to lessen the load when prices are high. **(T)**ransitory minded investors accept the changes (taxation, fiscal policy, monetary policy, secular changes, the internet of things, demographics, et cetera), roll with them, and are flexible and adaptive. **(A)**ge and awareness matter. Invest your age in bonds. **(R)**otate and rebalance into uncorrelated asset classes.

One of my clients was a professor who taught at my alma mater, Palm Beach Atlantic University. She was a saver and a virtuous lady. As a teacher, she never made a high salary, yet she regularly invested $25 weekly into mutual funds. By the time she was ready to retire, her liquid net worth exceeded $1 million. Again, I am not asserting that a vast sum of money is what honors a person (although I used to); it is the behavior that accompanies that accumulation that I do find dignifying. Saving requires moderation. Saving regularly is an act of discipline. Healthy habits derived from systematic saving directly translate into savvy business and personal decisions. Discipline in this context is about self-preservation and living life abundantly, untethered by possessions.

Minimalism

Have you ever gone shopping to purchase something, but chose not to the exact moment you walked up to the checkout counter? You delayed your immediate gratification by not purchasing the item, even though you had the extra funds. That's how it works. We live in the age of consumerism where a 30 year old living in America is hit with over 2,000 advertisements a day! It is an all-out ambush: billboards, internet, television, radio, movies, sporting events, concerts and more. Everywhere we turn we are bombarded by advertisements trying to seduce us into spending our money. Speak out by saving, and just say no!

Less is more. Facebook's Mark Zuckerberg, one of the ten richest people in the world, wears the same type of t-shirt nearly every day. Why? Because he wants his head to be clear of all the clutter that comes from unimportant decision making. If a gazillionaire like Zuckerberg is managing his finances frugally, as are Warren Buffett and countless others, so can we.

The Pareto principle (also known as the 80/20 rule or the law of the vital few) states that we use twenty percent of our belongings, wear twenty percent of our clothing, and perform twenty percent of our activities, eighty percent of the time. So, why do we need to have all this excess? How many pairs of pants, shoes, purses, and accessories are sufficient? Many of us do not know where all our belongings are in the first place, which leads to repurchasing the item(s) again.

The success of less begins this moment. Start by discarding something right away; it isn't hard to do. Schedule 10 to 15 minutes into your week to remove and discard some things. In a month's time there will be a noticeable improvement, in a year, even more. Minimalism is an ultramarathon that leads to clarity and contentment. It is a process toward a vibrant existence. The success of less is one of the best steps toward achieving permanent *Financial Fitness.*

There's an ancient proverb that says, "The best time to plant a tree was 20 years ago. The second best time is now." There are numerous books, videos, and articles on tidying and minimalism. Minimalism to me isn't an orthodoxy; it is an ideal. Keep less, focus more. It takes restraint to make the best decision. Making the right decision is well worth it, because making the right decision makes the decision maker happy. Start saving and plant that money tree today!

CHAPTER 14:

Success Shortcuts

"Proximity is power!"
—Tony Robbins

Congratulations on making it to this point in the book! Whether you arrived at this chapter by reading it cover-to-cover or jumping around is irrelevant. What's important is that by reaching this chapter it shows that you are willing to go the distance and dig deeper for answers that will improve your life. Ours is a world full of conventions. From the very start, our lives are molded with rules, guidelines, standards, and benchmarks that are deemed essential to win the prize. The prize is whatever makes our lives fulfilling, privately and professionally. Society's conventions seem to have an ironclad way of casting us all in the same mold, even though we are uniquely different. Conventions are neither good nor bad. They are a means for us to functionally coexist. However, there are times when conventions should be thrown out the door and replaced by a new set of directives.

Acquisitions

All my life I heard folks say things like, "There are no shortcuts to success" or "Climbing the corporate ladder is achieved one rung at a time." The list of clichés goes on. It's true that being accepted into an Ivy League school requires top grades and a lot of hard work; it's esteemable, but no guarantee to fame and fortune.

In fact, *The Crimson,* Harvard's news portal, recently published that median family income (two or more people) for Harvard undergraduates is $168,800. Well, I made Bs, had a ton of fun at my small liberal arts college, and have done okay just the same. If I can do it, anyone can. And yes, there are shortcuts!

For a business to simply survive, it has to grow. For a business to thrive, it must continue to expand. How is this accomplished? There are two primary ways to grow a business: organically one customer at a time or by mergers and acquisitions, in which customer growth is exponential. Most successful companies employ both strategies. Is there a shortcut? You bet there is; it is in buying existing profitable companies. An accretive acquisition can instantly springboard an ongoing company. For the intrepid soul who wants to start their own business, the act of buying an existing one is uncommon. The three reasons mostly cited for not buying an existing business at the onset or to accelerate the growth of a current business are: 1) I don't have the capital to purchase it; 2) I never considered the idea before; 3) I don't have enough experience to run a larger business. Each reason is valid.

My cousin David Dickens, a hardworking, talented business person, asked me how he could triple his income. He was aware that conventional methods would require him to make three times as many calls to get three times as many sales, but he knew it would be impossible to work three times as many hours. He had already tried to increase the output per each customer, i.e. going after the big client, but he felt loyal to his small accounts and gained a sense of security from the greater number of clients. I proposed that David try to buy out one of his competitors. I reminded David that all business owners have a fixed lifespan. At some point they have to turn the operation over to their family members, sell it to someone else, or close the business. I explained to him how I went to every trade show for small firms in my industry and introduced myself to as many owners as possible. I contacted vendors I knew and asked them to share my interest in buying or merging with other financial services firms. The strategy proved to be a windfall.

I believed in David's passion and integrity. I let him know that I would be open to funding and buying into the right deal. He was excited to have my endorsement and ready to move forward. I'm pleased to tell you that he found, negotiated, and bought a competitor within 30 minutes of his home. Within a few years, he tripled his income. As for my capital commitment, it never happened. The seller of the business took a reasonable down payment from David and provided owner financing for the bulk of the purchase. David made payments for the purchase from the acquired business' cash flow. That's what I call a win-win situation.

I have completed multiple deals over the past 20 years, and knock-on-wood, they've served me well. I've found that businesses that have been around for years often have exceptional employees; my company is a living example. Running a business successfully requires focus, commitment, the desire to be the best, and emotional intelligence. I aspire to the truism, "Nothing ventured, nothing gained." But there are caveats. Capitalism is the highly competitive game that never sleeps. There are real risks in running a business; it isn't for everyone. However, if you are the type of individual that relishes in the intensity of it all, being an entrepreneur could be your calling.

O.P.M.

The way to bring an idea to the forefront is by using other people's money or O.P.M. The consensus view espouses, "Cash is king." Here again, I take the variant view and argue, "Ideas are king." How much money is sitting in banks right now earning virtually zip? According to *Business Insider*, $50 trillion is sitting in cash. That's a ton of money ready to invest in the right idea. Before embarking on a new idea or venture, it is imperative to examine the idea thoroughly. Facebook was just an idea until Mark Zuckerberg and Eduardo Saverin brought it to life. Amazon was supposed to be an online book store, but Jeff Bezos had other ideas. Ideas prompt us to either do something with them or not. Warren Buffett bought a textile company and swears it was a bad idea. Mr. Buffett is an ideas guy and has utilized money from others to bring his ideas to life. In turn, investors who funded these ideas became very rich.

Successful entrepreneurs dwell in an ideas world. Ideas that make a positive impact in others' lives are being developed every minute. Bezos' vision is for Amazon to become the go to utility for everything for everyone. Tesla and SpaceX CEO, Elon Musk, aspires to put a colony of people on Mars. Each of us has our own ideas, notions and concepts; I bet one of those ideas could be a money maker. So, what does it take to bring these incredible ideas to life? It takes human ingenuity and capital. Successful entrepreneurs use other people's money. What if you don't have any venture capital? You need to find it. There are citizens in every community that have an abundance of money to invest. For the most part, they've built their wealth by being fair in their dealings, good stewards of their time, and practical with their capital resources. And, they took risk. They invest in startups, residential property, structures, existing companies and people. If you are speculating in real estate, building a new business or purchasing an ongoing enterprise, utilizing other people's money is powerful. People with money to invest have been shrewd at making it, investing it, and saving it. If they are willing and choose to invest in your innovative idea, they will be glad to share their insight and experience to help you succeed. If you have a well thought out idea with passion and energy behind it, get it funded. With $50 trillion lying around looking for a home, there is no shortage of interested parties.

Proximity is Power

A few years ago I attended Tony Robbins' Business Mastery conference. If you've ever attended one of Tony's events, you know that it is high impact, high tempo. When I was a younger man, I purchased Robbins' *Personal Power* cassettes and took ownership of the content; since then, I've been a fan. During the conference Robbins used the phrase, "Proximity is Power." I loved it! Immediately, it resonated with me. Why? Because I've witnessed in my own life the power of being around the right people: people of influence; winners at the next level; minds that have seen more than me; and individuals who have more experience. I'm talking about open-minded and open-hearted people who are interested in making the world a better place. Not only do these successful people have insight and knowledge, they invariably have a network of other like-minded leaders with various backgrounds and skill sets. All it takes to enter the proximity is power world is to identify and meet with a role model. Try it!

In Napoleon Hill's book, *Think and Grow Rich,* he introduces the idea of a mastermind alliance. Mastermind groups intertwine people's collective reasoning by way of listening, sharing, and caring. I am honored to be a founding member of the Elite Gentlemen's Organization or EGO for short. EGO is a small group of diverse personalities, professions, and faiths, whose societal differences outweigh our similarities. EGO has become a trusting bond of brothers absent of judgment and condemnation. None of our members had ever been in a mastermind alliance prior. We formed our club on the fly. EGOs motto: Inspire others and achieve greatness (however defined). During each mastermind meeting, we listen to each member share their current situation and goals, and we discuss how we can make our dreams come true. Each meeting, we write down three things we want to accomplish in the next month and the group holds us accountable. We eat and drink together, share our strengths, weaknesses and dreams with one another, and grow together. The message is simple: proximity is power.

"And will you succeed? Yes!
You will indeed! (98 and ¾ percent guaranteed.)"
—Dr. Seuss

How It Works:

Coach Lisa's Schedule	
Saturday	15 miles on the bridge: Power walk (PW) up and run down hard; then run good pace up and easy down; repeat for 15 miles. If you feel good run another 5 miles easy at 9:30-10:30 pace. Stretch.
Sunday	PW tire pull for 4 miles, then dump the tire; run easy to good pace for another 6 miles at 8:85-9:30 pace. Yoga.
Monday	Take the day off or swim 1,000 meters.
Tuesday	7 miles: run easy for 2 miles at 9:15-9:30 pace; then for 5 miles do 1/2 mile hard at 7:30 pace and 1/2 mile easy. Weights.
Wednesday	Bike up to 25 miles with your group. Extra exercises.
Thursday	8 miles: 2 miles at 8:50-9 pace; then alternate 1 mile at 7:30 pace and 1 mile at 8:50 pace for 6 miles. Yoga. Weights.
Friday	Swim for 1,000 meters. Extra exercises.
Saturday	20 miles on flat road: the first 10 miles at 9:15-9:20 pace; then 10 miles at 8:40-8:45 pace. Stretch.
Sunday	PW tire pull for 4 miles; then run 6 miles at 8:30 pace. Extra exercises.
Monday	Take the day off or yoga.
Tuesday	8 miles: run 2 miles easy at 9:30-10 pace; 1 mile hard at 7:15 pace, 1 mile easy as you feel like. Extra exercises.
Wednesday	Repeat last Wed.
Thursday	7 miles: run easy for 2 miles at 9:15-9:30 pace. Goal is 8 x 1/4 mile at 7-7:10 pace, followed by 1/4 mile easy at 9:30-10 pace. Extra exercises.
Friday	Swim for 1,000 meters. Extra exercises.
Extra Exercises	Burpees 2 x 20; wall sit 3 x 1 minute; planks 3 x 1 minute; jumping jacks 2 x 30; toe raises 2 x 20; mountain climbers 2 x 20; squats 2 x 20; lunges 2 x 20; high knees 2 x 20; push-ups 3 x 15-20; 3 x 25 sit-ups; jump rope.
Weights	Dumbbells 25 lbs squat thrusts 3 x 20; curls 3 x 20; triceps 3 x 20

Weekly Ritual:

"The quality of your life is in direct relationship to the quality of your habits and rituals."
—Stan Jacobs.

Week at a Glance

	Mon	Tue	Wed	Thu	Fri	Sat	Sun
6:00 AM	–	Speed Run	Bike	Tempo Run	Easy Run	Long Run	Tire Pull & Run
7:00 AM	Work Begins	–	–	Hot Yoga	–	–	–
8:00 AM	–	Work Begins	Work Begins	Work Begins	Work Begins	–	Hot Yoga
10:00 AM	Dumbells at Desk	–	–	–	Dumbells at Desk	–	–
12:00 PM	Green Drink	Green Drink	Green Drink	Green Drink	Green Drink	Work Begins	–
5:00 PM	Work Ends	Work Ends	Work Ends	Work Ends	Work Ends	Work Ends	–
6:00 PM	Sauna	Extra Exercises	Meetings	Massage	–	–	Extra Exercises
7:00 PM	–	Meetings	–	Meetings	–	Free Time	Free Time
8:00 PM	Rest & Relaxation	–	Rest & Relaxation	–	Rest & Relaxation	–	–
9:00 PM	–	Rest & Relaxation	–	Rest & Relaxation	–	–	–

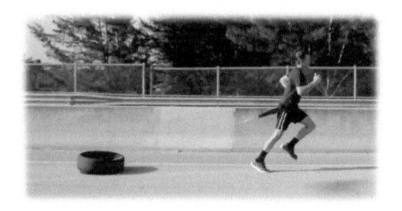

APPENDIX:
Frequently Used Sites and Apps
Organizing

✓ Evernote: If you want to get organized and work smarter, try Evernote. 200 million users rely on Evernote. I'm an Evernote Community Leader, here's a _free_ link. http://evernote.grsm.io/WilliamCorley
✓ TheTileApp.com: Helps you locate keys, purses, iPhone, etc.
✓ Hootsuite.com: Manage all social media in one place.

Learning

✓ MOOCs: Coursera, Udacity, Stanford Online and edX offer free online education. Each of these massive open online courses (MOOCs) offers free online learning at some of the best colleges and institutions. I have taken several classes from Coursera. My favorite was a free Sociology class at Princeton University.
✓ Reading: Audible (books); Natural Reader (text to speech); Pocket app (articles)

Shopping

✓ Amazon: Apply for the Amazon Credit Card and get 5% back on Amazon purchases.
✓ Jet.com: Get bargains on household items: toilet paper, laundry detergent (free shipping ≥ $35).

Savings

✓ Websites: Airbnb (lodging); Gasbuddy.com & Speedpass.com (gasoline); HomeExchange.com (vacation); Coupons.com, Currentcodes.com (coupons); Getaround.com, turo.com (car sharing & rental); JustPark (car parking); ThredUP.com (consignment shop); Freecycle.org (free stuff); Dinkytown.net (financial calculators); GoodRx.com (prescription prices); Swagbucks (earn gift cards); Gazelle.com (sell electronics); Senior Discounts (http://bit.ly/1S0m98w).

Meditation

✓ Headspace: To calm it all down, I've found Headspace ideal. I meditate 10 minutes a day.

ACKNOWLEDGMENTS

I would like to express my gratitude to the many people who were with me during my adventures throughout this book. Special thanks to my editor Jodi Weiss, MA, MFA, who enabled me through her guidance, know-how, patience, and persistence to bring this writing to fruition. William Corley III and Alaina De Renzo brought my story to life with their photography. Aileen Gallagher was my sounding board throughout this experience. Thanks also to my family and friends who provided support, offered comments, and allowed me to quote their remarks.